PEEK-A-BOOB
Uncovering Breast Cancer

SHELLEY MALICOTE STUTCHMAN

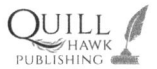

QUILL HAWK PUBLISHING

Copyright © 2024 by Shelley Malicote Stutcham

All rights reserved.

This book or parts thereof may not be reproduced in any form, stored in a retrieval system, or transmitted in any form by any means, electronic, mechanical, photocopy, recording, or otherwise, without prior written permission of the author or publisher, except as provided by United States of America copyright law.

This book contains the opinions and ideas of its author and is based on the author's personal experience with breast cancer. Some of the views expressed are controversial. Readers are encouraged to consult with their doctors regarding their best treatment options.

The author is not engaged in rendering professional advice to the individual reader. The ideas contained in this book are solely for informational and educational purposes and should not be regarded as a substitute for professional medical treatment. Neither the author nor the publisher shall be liable or responsible for any loss or damage allegedly arising from any information or suggestions in this book.

While the author has made every effort to provide accurate internet addresses and information at the time of publication, neither the publisher nor the author assumes any responsibility for errors or for changes that occur after publication.

Cover photo by Ralph Bernhardt

Edited by Robyn Conley, The Book Doctor

ISBN: 979-8-9900749-4-1 (Paperback)

ISBN: 979-8-9900749-5-8 (Hardback)

Library of Congress Control Number: 2024915556

Quill Hawk Publishing

Contents

Reviews	1
Dedication	4
Foreword	5
1. I HAVE WHAT	6
Cancer Post #1: Routine Mammogram: February 28th	7
Cancer Post #2: Breast Biopsy: March 7th	9
2. UNVEILING THE IDENTITY OF MY NEMESIS	14
Cancer Post #3: Portal: March 9th	15
Cancer Post #4: Plan of Action: March 11th	18
3. WANTING TO RUN	23
Cancer Post #5: Meeting the Surgeon: March 21st	24
Cancer Post #6: Bone Scan: March 23rd	27
Cancer Post #7: YouTube: March 24th	29
Cancer Post #8: Symptoms: March 28th	32
Cancer Post #9: Surgery Day: March 31st	34
Cancer Post #10: Recovery: April 5th	37
4. CONFRONTING THE SHADOW	40
Cancer Post #11: Freedom Beckons: April 7th	41

Cancer Post #12: Unveiling the Hidden Truth: April 10th ... 44

5. GOD WINKS ... 48

Cancer Post #13: Divine Whispers: April 12th ... 49

6. MY TUMOR'S ADVENTURE ... 53

Cancer Post #14: The BRCA Gene Test: April 18th ... 54

Cancer Post #15: Tale of My Vacationing Tumor: April 21st ... 56

Cancer Post #16: Chemotherapy: April 23rd ... 59

7. CORDING AND LYMPHEDEMA ... 66

Cancer Post #17: Hidden Hazards: April 30th ... 67

Cancer Post #18: Mysterious Disappearance of Symptoms: May 2nd ... 69

Cancer Post #19: Through the Lens: May 3rd ... 72

Cancer Post #20: Goodbye Sweets: May 4th ... 74

Cancer Post #21: Popeye and Olive Oyl: May 9th ... 76

8. LESSONS ... 79

Cancer Post #22: Revelations from the School of Life: May 13th ... 80

Cancer Post #23: Get Out of Town: May 20th ... 83

Cancer Post #24: Pause and Contemplate: May 29th ... 86

Cancer Post #25: Sisterly Chronicles: May 30th ... 89

9. RADIATION ... 93

Cancer Post #26: Trepidation and Joy: May 31st ... 94

Cancer Post #27: Eureka Moments: May 31st ... 96

Cancer Post #28: Reflections on the Eve of Surgery: May 31st ... 98

Cancer Post #29: Unexpected Workplace Prescription: June 1st ... 100

Cancer Post #30: Surgery was Fun: June 1st ... 102

Cancer Post #31: Gas: June 2nd ... 105

Cancer Post #32: Navigating Challenges with Valium: June 3rd ... 107

Cancer Post #33: Bathe, Saran Wrap, and The Total Woman: June 4th ... 110

Cancer Post #34: A Plush Haven: June 4th	112
Cancer Post #35: Fashion Armor for Modern Warriors: June 6th	114
Cancer Post #36: Two Down: June 6th	117
Cancer Post #37: Sex and Radiation: June 8th	120
10. BELLS	123
Cancer Post #38: Bells of Love and Resilience: June 10th	124
Cancer Post #39: TA: June 11th	126
11. WEDDING BELLS	129
Cancer Post #40: Love's Grand Overture: June 12th	130
Cancer Post #41: Daughters Unite: June 16th	132
Cancer Post #42: Feeling Groovy: June 17th	134
Cancer Post #43: No Sex: June 17th	136
12. MEN GET BREAST CANCER TOO	139
Cancer Post #44: Shadows of Breast Cancer: June 19th	140
13. THE SHIFT	143
Cancer Post #45: Airport Security: June 20th	144
Cancer Post #46: Shifting Priorities: June 24th	147
14. CHAINED	152
Cancer Post #47: Revving Up: June 26th	153
Cancer Post #48: Chained: June 27th	156
Cancer Post #49: My Second Day Back to Work: June 28th	158
15. HORMONE HORROR	161
Cancer Post #50: To Letrozole or not to Letrozole: June 30th	162
Cancer Post #51: Hilarious Hazards of Cancer: July 1st	165
Cancer Post #52: Thrills and Chills Hormone Horrors: July 8th	167
16. CELEBRATE	171
Cancer Post #53: One Month Cancer Free: July 10th	172

17. THE FINE LINE BETWEEN PARNOIAD AND CAUTIOUS	175
Cancer Post #54: Invisible Intruders: July 17th	176
Cancer Post #55: Sick Again: July 25th	178
Cancer Post #56: How Facebook Nurses Nailed It: July 26th	183
Cancer Post #57: Institute of Science: August 3rd	185
Cancer Post: #58: Self-Protection: August 5th	187
18. BREASTIES	190
Cancer Post #59: Besties in Battle: August 6th	191
19. FINDING BALANCE IN "JUST FEELING FAIR"	194
Cancer Post #60: MD Anderson: August 9th	195
20. GUARDIANS WITHIN: IMMUNE SYSTEM	198
Cancer Post #61: Goals: August 11th	199
21. OVERCOMING THE STRUGGLE OF SELF	204
Cancer Post #62: Mirror of Misgivings: August 12th	205
Cancer Post #63: Embracing the Sweat: August 13th	207
Cancer Post #64: Reclaiming My Dreams: August 15th	209
Cancer Post #65: The Bliss of Feeling Good: August 19th	211
Cancer Post #66: Mindset Mastery: August 21st	213
22. LADY PARTS AND WEIGHT GAIN	216
Cancer Post #67: Sacred Spaces: August 22nd	217
Cancer Post #68: Battling the Bulge: August 23rd	219
Cancer Post #69: Work That Body: August 30th	221
23. TRIALS AND DECISIONS	224
Cancer Post #70: Clinical Trials: August 28th	225
24. CANCER WINS WHEN	229
Cancer Post #71: Understanding When Cancer Wins: September 6th	230
25. DOWN THERE	233

Cancer Post #72: A Continuation: September 7th	234
Cancer Post #73: Smart Alec: September 9th	237
Cancer Post #74: Three-Month Cancer Free Party: September 10th	239
Cancer Post #75: Staring Cancer in The Faith: September 12th	241
Cancer Post #76: Today's Momentous Journey: September 21st	243
Cancer Post #77: Weighing In: September 23rd	245
Cancer Post #78: Passing the Torch: September 25th	247
Cancer Post #79: The Biopsy's Revelation: September 27th	249
Cancer Post #80: The Doctor's Call: September 28th	252
26. BODY REMODELING	255
Cancer Post #81: Breast Size: October 5th	256
Cancer Post #82: A Deceased Woman's Breast: October 8th	258
27. ANXIETY TRIGGERS	261
Cancer Post #83: Well, this is Scary: October 9th	262
Cancer Post #84: Rash: October 11th	264
Cancer Post #85: Swimming Suit Anxiety: October 16th	266
28. GHOSTING	269
Cancer Post #86: Vanishing Act: October 27th	270
29. FOGGY BRAIN	273
Cancer Post #87: Echoes of Forgetfulness: November 6th	274
Cancer Post #88: Try to Remember: November 9th	278
Cancer Post #89: Skin Cancer Side Effect: November 13th	280
Cancer Post #90: Echoes of Kinship: November 18th	282
Cancer Post #91: No More: November 25th	286
30. TWENTY THOUSAND DOLLAR BOOBS	289
Cancer Post #92: Reconstruction: November 28th	290
Cancer Post #93: Random Thoughts: November 29th	292

Cancer Post #94: The Last Incision: November 30th	294
Cancer Post #95: Perky: December 1st	296
Cancer Post #96: The Heavy Burden: December 2nd	298
Cancer Post #97: Peak-A-Boob: December 3rd	300
Cancer Post #98: Perseverance's Promise: December 5th	302
Cancer Post #99: Squeak: December 8th	304
Cancer Post #100: Bras: December 18th	306
31. MY HALLMARK CHRISTMAS	309
Cancer Post #101: Christmas: December 26th	310
32. THE WHY'S	314
Cancer Post #102: I Got Cancer Because: December 28th	315
Cancer Post #103: The Gastric Gambit: January 2nd	320
33. INSURANCE, MEDICARE, PAYMENTS…OH MY	323
Cancer Post #104: Policy of Fury: January 6th	324
Cancer Post #105: Exploring Medicare: January 8th	327
34. HEARTBREAK LINKED TO BREAST CANCER	330
Cancer Post #106: Sick Heart: January 9th	331
35. I BOOKED A CRUISE AND OTHER RANDOM THINGS	334
Cancer Post #107: Seven Months: January 10th	335
Cancer Post #108: Cruise: January 13th	337
Cancer Post #109: Sunscreen Lotions: January 18th	339
Cancer Post #110: Slimming Solutions: January 20th	341
Cancer Post #111: Hand Power: January 23rd	343
Cancer Post #112: Body Dysmorphic Disorder: January 24th	345
36. NO FAVORS	348
Cancer Post #113: Don't Ask Me: January 30th	349
37. HAPPY BIRTHDAY	355

Cancer Post #114: Joyous Anniversary of Birth: February 3rd	356
Cancer Post #115: Nervous: February 6th	358
38. INTIMATE POSTS	361
Cancer Post #116: Potentially Controversial: February 8th	362
Cancer Post #117: My Son Has Cancer: February 9th	364
39. MUSIC AND WORDS	368
Cancer Post #118: Music of Joel Sebring: March 4th	369
Cancer Post #119: Unraveling Meanings: March 5th	372
40. RECURRENCE	377
Cancer Post #120: Stand by your Friend: March 27th	378
41. DOWN AND DIRTY	381
Cancer Post #121: Sexy Challenges: March 29th	382
42. LITTLE GIRL'S THOUGHTS ABOUT BREAST CANCER	386
Cancer Post #122: Little Girls are Listening: April 11th	387
43. THE CRUISE	389
Cancer Post #123: Seafaring: April 24th	390
44. MAN TO MAN	393
Cancer Post #124: Neil Talks to the Guys: May 2nd	394
Acknowledgements	401
About the author	402
Thank you	403
Unveiling the Soul of Quotes	404
CITATIONS FOR QUOTES	416
CITATIONS FOR RESEARCH	424

Reviews

"In this book about surviving breast cancer, Stutchman captures the fragility of life through her expressive, beautiful writing. As she navigates through her often-poignant journey, you can feel her fears, her brief doubt of faith, and her uncertainties about her future. The love and importance of her family is ever present. I was delighted to see the chapter written by her sister. Her candidness about her intimacy with her husband spoke to a real situation many may not have considered. While it is just one person's experience, the author's presentation brings the reader a feeling of candid reality. There is truly a valuable and possibly humorous take away from her story. I recommend this book for any woman, at any age, who is diagnosed with breast cancer."

—Jodi Cooper, Susan G. Komen® Volunteer-Event Committee Chairperson

"Three of the most frightening words one can ever hear are: YOU HAVE CANCER. Medical books and journals provide all kinds of facts and figures, such as staging, grading, treatments, outcomes, and survival rates, which are all important. In this well-written book, Shelley Malicote Stutchman shares her feelings and experiences from the first suspicious mammogram to ringing the cancer-free bell with her fiancé. This was followed by the whys, the what ifs, and worries of cancer recurrence. Shelley speaks of hope and faith in that order and gives a wonderful definition of both. Her journey in the diagnosis and treatment of breast cancer is both enlightening, very personal, and scary for anyone who has breast cancer or any other type of cancer. Shelley explains how her treatment was multifaceted to include physical, mental, social, emotional, and spiritual experiences. In the last chapter, the male perspective is given. Early diagnosis and treatment are the best keys to survival in this all too common and dreaded disease.

This book teaches one that knowledge is power and suggests that one should not be hubris while navigating through available treatment options."

—Michael B. Scott, D.O., Physician and Surgeon, Retired

"In her raw, honest, and empowering memoir "Peek a Boob," Shelley takes readers on her personal journey battling breast cancer. With candid humor and heartfelt emotion, she provides a source of solidarity for her "Pink Sisters" also facing this disease.

While chronicling her own tests, treatments, and experiences, Shelley covers a wealth of practical information that makes this book an educational resource as well. She directly addresses the difficult and often unasked questions that arise, explaining medical realities in easy-to-understand terminology. As a registered nurse, I found Shelley's research and insights to be a valuable guide for breast cancer patients and their loved ones.

What sets "Peek a Boob" apart is Shelley's empathetic yet empowering tone throughout. Each chapter offers emotional support and sisterhood for readers going through their own cancer battles. Her ability to share uncomfortable truths through the lens of her inspiring resilience is remarkable."

—DanaTramba, R.N., Author of Making Peace with the Pieces of My Life (www.Dandystories.com)

"The day Shelley Stutchman was diagnosed with Breast Cancer was the day her journey began. The author takes the reader through her fears and misgivings. She also talks about all the research completed to help guide her decision-making as to the medical care needed for her survival. Her courage and tenacity stand out for all who have the privilege of reading her story. Shelley Stutchman puts her heart and soul into this book and utilizes it as a tool for those going down the same path."

—Jacquelyne Hume RNBSN, (Retired)

When I first met Shelley Malicote Stutchman, I knew that I had met a friend for life. She was marketing for a hospice company, and I was a case manager for a small rural hospital. She had all the qualities of a great friend, and she was a brilliant conversationalist. Our friendship was made deeper by our ability to share life experiences.

The ability to share her life experiences is a huge part of her writing this book, "Peek-A-Boob." The reader will find this book not only informative and inspirational but also humorous and emotional. The writings will be helpful for those who have found themselves on their own journey with breast cancer, as well as their family and friends. I feel that it will also be helpful for those navigating the medical community.

I love that with each chapter, Shelley shares:

• Her cancer research on the current topic

• An uplifting quote for the day

• A space for writing thoughts/questions

Shelley also shares tips about her procedures and what to expect and how to help the process. As a medical professional, I feel an important aspect of the book is that she breaks down medical terminology - how to pronounce it and the meaning of the word. A patient's ability to understand medical terminolog yallows them to understand, process, and use health information to make decisions about their health."

—Debra Hightower, AND, RN

For all the brave women who have faced a breast cancer diagnosis, this book is dedicated to you. Through my personal journey and heartfelt words, I hope to offer guidance through difficult emotions, education through researching cancer topics, inspiration through uplifting quotes, and clarity on treatment options. May PEEK-A-BOOB serve as a source of strength in overcoming this disease. This is the book I longed for when I first heard the words, "You have breast cancer."

With special thanks and love to:

Cameraman (Neil) Johnson, my loving and groovy husband.

Ginger Stutchman and Ryan Stutchman, my children.

Horace Stutchman, my wasbund.

Natalie Gustafon and Melissa Fales, my bonus daughters.

Willow LaMunyon, my always supportive sister.

Luana Ash, my friend and constant researcher.

Foreword

The doctor's words hit me like a freight train, shattering my sense of security and hurling me into a terrifying new reality, "You have Breast Cancer." The very word, cancer, filled me with dread and sent chills down my spine. I scrolled through Facebook, seeking solace in the stories of others, and through their narratives, I found the courage to share my journey with this devastating disease.

From surgeries and treatments to getting married and going on a honeymoon, my life became a chaotic whirlwind of fighting cancer. And amidst it all, I promised myself, God, and the Universe I would be open about my journey, hoping to give strength to others facing similar battles.

When I hit "post" on my first Facebook update announcing my breast cancer diagnosis, doubt crept in - was it too personal? Soon enough, I received my answer as messages poured in from strangers who found comfort and inspiration in my words.

As I share my story, I hope that it will bring comfort to those struggling, remind them of the power of vulnerability and community, and inspire others to find their strength and courage in the face of adversity. This is not just my story—it is the story of all those who have been touched by cancer and the resilience that lies within us all.

—Shelley Malicote Stutchman, Survivor

Chapter One

I HAVE WHAT

Cancer Post #1: Routine Mammogram: February 28th

My cell rang ten minutes before my shift ended, and I could begin the weekend. The person spoke in a composed manner, "I'm calling from the breast center to inform you that an irregularity was detected on your mammogram." She added, "We need to schedule you for an ultrasound."

For a fleeting moment, my mind went blank, and all rational thought escaped me. A crushing weight pressed down on my chest, squeezing the air out of my lungs like a deflating balloon. I remained frozen in my office chair, unable to process the news. I reminded myself to stay calm and just breathe. I needed to gather my thoughts before they spiraled out of control.

"How about Monday, March 7th at 9 a.m.? Does that fit into your schedule?" she asked.

I frantically scanned through my jam-packed work calendar. Commitments and responsibilities filled every second of my days, but none seemed as pressing as my current health situation. "I'll be there," I answered.

The phone call ended, leaving my mind screaming with the worst possibilities. My fingers trembled when I redialed the testing center's number again, only to hear a recorded message explaining that if this was an emergency, to call 911. If not an emergency, call back during their regular business hours. In my head, alarms blared while the rest of the world carried on as if nothing was wrong. A desperate prayer escaped from me, pleading I wouldn't be another woman in the battle against breast cancer.

The statistics weighed heavily on my mind. One in eight women...that was a lot. Both my mother and sister had fought against breast cancer. My sister survived, but my mother died. It couldn't happen to all three of us, could it? The odds had to be in my favor. Right?

I denied my illness, refusing to acknowledge the possibility of cancer, believing it was only a harmless fibroid. I promised myself to keep the situation private until I received my test results, only confiding in my fiancé.

Yet I worried. The weeks of exhaustion suddenly made sense. As soon as I got home from work, I'd curl up on the couch beneath the blanket I'd left unfolded days before. Reaching for the TV remote took more effort than I wanted. Despite all these signs, I kept pushing them aside with false logic; after all, at sixty-seven, I figured working a full-time job might be more taxing on me than I realized. I could have retired a year ago, but I got satisfaction from my job. Surely, hard work and my age created this fatigue, not cancer.

To ease my worries, I decided to research Google about callbacks after a mammogram.

***

Internet Research:

https://www.cancer.org/cancer/breast-cancer/screening-tests-and-early-detection/mammograms/getting-called-back-after-a-mammogram.htm

Getting called back after a screening mammogram is fairly common, and it doesn't mean you have breast cancer. In fact, fewer than 1 in 10 women called back for more tests are found to have cancer. Often, it just means more mammograms or other tests (such as an ultrasound) need to be done to get a closer look at an area of concern.

***

This piece of information from the web sounded promising. Whenever I'm stressed, I turn to research and quotes. The following quote helped get me through the week.

Today's Quote:

"Half the worry in the world is caused by people trying to make decisions before they have sufficient knowledge on which to base a decision."

—Herbert E. Hawkes

A Note to You:

Your breast cancer diagnosis slams you to the ground like a hard slap in the face. The questions, emotions, and possible spiritual battles overwhelm your senses and plunge you into a deep ocean of the unknown. This book takes your hand and guides you out of this abyss, with each post providing insight into my journey with breast cancer and research from the finest medical institutions and studies. There are inspiring quotes for days when hope fades away. I'm here with you every step of the way as we become more than just pink sisters - we become survivors.

Cancer Post #2: Breast Biopsy: March 7th

Cancerous thoughts crept into my mind repeatedly with each waking hour, I knew letting those contemplations takeover would not benefit me, so I tried to maintain control over my negative thoughts. I rationalized many women were called back for mammograms because of fibroids or dense breast tissue. My fiancé, Neil, reassured me with this same logic, telling me not to worry until the tests revealed the reason for the abnormal mammogram. With a gentle expression, he said, "We're both getting older, and our bodies are changing."

I struggled to keep the news about my test results a secret from my coworkers. However, every fiber of my being yearned for their reassurance. I wanted to hear them tell me the suspicious spot on my scan was nothing to worry about. When struggling to stay afloat, validation and support could feel like a life vest. I didn't want to raise any alarms when there was no fire. I threw myself into my job with renewed vigor, determined to keep busy and productive to drown out the negative thoughts consuming me. Each day became a race against time, a desperate attempt to outrun the fear and uncertainty plaguing me.

I walked into my boss's office on Thursday, took a deep breath and explained the situation. She listened intently as I spoke, occasionally nodding in understanding. My deceased mother's advice to never shed tears in the workplace echoed in my mind. "Crying at work portrays vulnerability and hinders progress," she would say.

Despite the familiar words echoing in my mind, tears threatened to spill from my eyes. But I held them back, determined to maintain composure. When I finished speaking, my boss thanked me for letting her know and assured me there would be no issues with arriving late on Monday.

Saturday and Sunday seemed to blur together as I drowned myself in episode after episode on Netflix, surrounded by empty tubs of ice cream and wrappers of chocolate. My scale revealed a gain of three pounds in just two days. My coping mechanism spiraled out of control. TV and sweets provided me with the same distraction as alcohol to an alcoholic. But how could I resist when these vices were the only things calming my inner turmoil?

Monday morning arrived, and I tried to cover the dark circles under my eyes with makeup. No amount of concealer could hide the exhaustion and fear etched into my face. I visualized the doctor telling me the spot was benign and that I wouldn't need to return for another year. In my unconventional yet spiritually aligned perspective, I firmly believed manifesting a clear and precise vision could bring it to fruition.

Neil and I drove to the breast center in silence, which was unusual for us. We usually chattered non-stop, but the gravity of the situation made it difficult to choose the right words. Luckily, we found an excellent parking spot, which felt like a sign that everything would turn out fine.

When we entered the empty waiting room, I felt oddly agitated. We took a seat in the plush chairs. In just a few minutes, a nurse appeared at the door, scanning the entire area before announcing my name. Who else could it be? I wondered if she was a few fries short of a happy meal.

We stepped into the sterile atmosphere of the exam room, filled with various machines and equipment, an examination table, one chair, and the strong scent of disinfectant. The nurse assured me that my partner Neil could stay by my side. It made me hurt for the women who have to go through this experience alone. A technician entered and handed me a cape. She instructed me to remove my blouse and bra and put the opening of the cape in the front. The staff's kindness and attentiveness were a source of comfort.

I draped the soft, flowing pink cape around my shoulders. With a playful twirl, I pranced in front of Neil, the fabric billowing behind me. With a coy smile, I asked, "Do you find me alluring?"

His lips curved upwards in a small but genuine smile. The only smile we shared that day.

The technician re-entered the room with a tray full of medical supplies. She donned blue rubber gloves before lightly dabbing my bare breast with a cold, sterile antiseptic solution. I shivered. A few minutes later, a woman with a slender frame, a flawless complexion, and an unreadable expression entered the room. "Hello, I'm the doctor on your case today," she said while applying a sticky gel to both of my breasts.

She never took her eyes off the monitor as she slid the paddle in methodical circles over my skin. She paused and focused more deliberately when she reached my left side, sliding the paddle over the same spot multiple times. I couldn't decipher any clues from her face about what she may have found. After what felt like an eternity, she turned to us and said, "I need to do a biopsy."

I struggled to utter, "When?"

My mind and heart were at odds, torn between wanting to know the answer and fearing what it might be. Part of me wanted to run away from the truth, but another part was desperate to face it head-on.

"Now."

That single word hung in the air.

My eyes met Neil's, and I noticed a glistening tear he failed to conceal. It hit me our plans for the future were now uncertain, cast into the shadows of fear and doubt. If the biopsy results returned positive for cancer, would he still be there for me? We exchanged nervous glances. Our unspoken bond as lovers felt both strong and fragile. We nodded in unison with the doctor's words, trying to reassure ourselves everything would be okay.

The doctor shared the ultrasound results but couldn't confirm cancer without additional tests. Her language seemed more legal than medical.

The technological assistant presented an array of medical supplies, including needles, wipes, bottles of liquids, containers for specimens, gauze, and other items whose purposes I couldn't discern. The doctor selected a needle and extracted a liquid from one of the bottles, clarifying that she was administering a numbing agent to the biopsy area. As they exited to allow the medication to take effect, Neil and I exchanged uneasy glances. Searching for a topic of conversation, we landed on the stock market's decline that day. Despite our efforts, a sense of unease hung over us.

After about ten minutes, the doctor and aide returned, ready to begin the procedure. The doctor collected two samples from my breast using a syringe. I felt a little pain, uncomfortable, but bearable. I sat up, assuming the tests were finished. The doctor said, "We need to perform a biopsy on a couple of lymph nodes under your arm."

Feeling confused, I asked, "Why?"

"Some of the lymph nodes are concerning."

The doctor neglected to mention the excruciating agony that would accompany the biopsy under my arm. As the needle pierced my skin, I let out a gut-wrenching scream, feeling as if all the torments of hell were being inflicted upon me simultaneously. And yet, I could do nothing but grit my teeth and endure as she extracted samples from another area underneath my arm.

The pain subsided immediately when the doctor completed the biopsy. The tech aide meticulously wrapped my tender flesh in soft gauze and gently placed a soothing ice pack on it. "Make sure to take some Tylenol when you get home," she advised, her voice filled with sympathy.

"When will you get the results?" I asked the doctor.

"Around four days," she answered.

So began our new routine of being placed in a constant state of urgency, rushing to get tested and then waiting and waiting for the results.

I stared at my phone and tried to find the right words to tell my boss I was in too much pain to come back to work. I hated letting her down, and I needed the money. Reluctantly, I typed out the text and hit send, feeling guilty as I did.

On the drive home, Neil turned to me, "Is there anything you want or need?"

I paused, "Just a vanilla malt from Braums."

***

Internet Research:

Breast biopsy – Mayo Clinic

The results of a breast biopsy can show whether the area in question is breast cancer or if it's not cancerous. The pathology report from the breast biopsy can help your doctor determine whether you need additional surgery or other treatment.

***

Today's Quote:

"Trust yourself. You've survived a lot, and you'll survive whatever is coming."

—Robert Tew

A Note to You:

During your biopsy, make sure you have someone there with whom you feel comfortable seeing your breasts. Have them take notes or record the doctor's instructions on your phone. And afterward, don't forget to take care of yourself. Ask a friend to stay with you and treat you like the queen you are. You deserve some pampering.

PEEK-A-BOOB

NOTES AND THOUGHTS

CHAPTER TWO

UNVEILING THE IDENTITY OF MY NEMESIS

Cancer Post #3: Portal: March 9th

When I arrived at work the next day, a dull ache throbbed in my chest and left underarm. I tried to act normal. Despite my efforts to appear calm and collected, my coworkers asked about my health. Not wanting to reveal the uncertain results of my tests, I brushed it off as simply undergoing routine medical procedures.

After a grueling day at work, I trudged to the home Neil and I shared, my shoulders heavy. The setting sun streaming through my upstairs office window put harsh rays onto my computer screen. With a deep sigh, I switched on the monitor. I mindlessly scrolled through Facebook, pausing to admire photos of grilled chicken and vegetables posted by friends. But despite the distractions, my thoughts were consumed by checking the lab results on my patient portal. Like two opposing forces perched upon my shoulders, an angel and devil tugged at my conscience - one urging me to satisfy my curiosity while the other warned against jumping to conclusions without consulting the doctor first. I struggled between giving in to my anxious thoughts or heeding the advice of my inner voice.

I logged into my patient portal and clicked on the test results. I couldn't believe what I saw: "malignancy of the left female breast." Those words stared back at me, cold and unfeeling. Dread washed over me as I read on, seeing phrases like "unspecified estrogen receptor status" and "unspecified site of breast." Those few sentences on a digital page forever altered my life and future.

I looked at the lab report in disbelief. I had cancer? The thought alone should have brought me to tears, but instead, a strange sense of calm settled over me. When I typed the words into Google, a million thoughts raced. How would I break this news to Neil? How could I possibly cope with such a devastating diagnosis? I was torn between denial and acceptance, unsure of how to handle this conflicting mix of emotions.

I feverishly searched through endless medical jargon until I stumbled upon the interpretation of my lab results from the almighty Dr. Google. I found a simplified definition that my panicked mind could grasp. What is a malignant neoplasm? A malignant neoplasm (NEE-oh-plaz-um) is another term for a cancerous tumor. The term "neoplasm" refers to abnormal growth of tissue. The term "malignant" means the tumor is cancerous and is likely to spread (metastasize) beyond its point of origin.

I headed towards Neil's office with purpose, leaving my computer behind. Despite the news, I maintained my composure. As I neared his door, I could see him hunched over his computer screen with a look of frustration. "Hi, sweetie. I'm feeling a bit overwhelmed with all the political noise lately. It's exhausting trying to keep up with everything."

Neil sighed, running a hand through his hair. "I need to escape all this negativity and focus on positive things."

I sank into my usual comfy chair, unsure of what would unfold. "Wait a moment, I need to put in my hearing aids," Neil announced, catching the look of concern on my face.

Neil always inserted his hearing aids whenever we needed to talk. He ensured no part of our conversation would be lost, showing genuine kindness and care.

I shared the news of my test results in my portal. I wondered how I remained so calm; perhaps it was necessary to process the shocking results without completely breaking down.

Neil sank back into the supple leather of his brown chair and closed his eyes with a sigh, taking in the gravity of the situation. After what felt like an eternity, he opened them again and met my gaze. His blue eyes brimmed with warmth, determination, and love. "We are going to get through this," he said softly but firmly, never breaking eye contact.

The following day, my phone buzzed. It was the breast center. They scheduled an appointment for the next day. Was my cancer more serious than I had initially believed? I remembered how my other appointments were scheduled days or weeks in advance. This sudden urgency from the breast center left me shaken.

***

Internet Research:

Now What? First Steps After a Breast Cancer Diagnosis (healthgrades.com)

After your diagnosis, educate yourself so you can be confident about your decisions. Ask a close friend or family member to learn with you, attend your appointments, and be your advocate. A second set of ears and another point of view is invaluable when you are dealing with your new diagnosis.

***

Today's Quote:

"When you get diagnosed with cancer, there's such a sense of loneliness, but what we need to know as people going through this is that you're not alone."

—Christina Applegate

A Note to You:

My friend, I know that upon receiving the news of your diagnosis, it can feel as if the world has come to a standstill. You may be unable to think of anything else other than getting rid of this cancer from your body. Let me assure you everything you are feeling is perfectly normal for someone who has just been diagnosed. Take this time to reach out to a Facebook group or organization near you, where you can make connections with other pink sisters who have gone through the same experience.

Cancer Post #4: Plan of Action: March 11th

The nurse scheduled another appointment. But it sounded like a judge handing down a prison sentence to me.

Dread filled me at the thought of having to face my boss and colleagues with news of my medical condition. After working with them for four years, I considered my colleagues my second family. I knew their sweet expressions of sympathy and concern would make my diagnosis feel dreadfully real. I couldn't help feeling conflicted about sharing this news. A part of me wanted their support, while another part craved privacy during this difficult time.

I rapped my knuckles on my boss's door, and Cathy glanced up from her desk buried under a mountain of charts and tasks. Without hesitation, I spoke in a blunt, no-nonsense tone. "I have to take time off work. I've been diagnosed with cancer."

Without hesitation, she said, "Take whatever time you need."

I shared my concerns about taking time off for necessary treatments. Cathy listened patiently and understandingly. As a nurse, she knew the physical and emotional toll of these treatments and reassured me that it was okay to prioritize my health. She assured me my job would be waiting for me whenever I was ready to come back, and we would work together to ensure proper coverage during my absence. Her words brought a sense of comfort in what seemed like an overwhelming situation.

I forced a smile, but it came off as insincere. As a veteran in the marketing and sales industry, I knew better than to burden others with my personal problems. My training taught me to listen attentively and empathize with others, regardless of my struggles. My world may have been falling apart, but I kept up a façade, hiding my internal struggles behind a practiced expression.

My boss was a lifesaver, understanding my situation and accommodating me. My heart ached knowing many other cancer patients struggle with the added burden of balancing work and health. I prayed for other companies to see the light and prioritize the well-being of their employees.

I shared the news with my colleagues during lunch. They asked how to help me. I told them, "Please, let things feel normal. Let's talk about everything and nothing during our lunch break like always."

Linda, who managed our office, shifted the topic and shared a heartwarming moment of her grandson's cute actions captured on video. She passed her phone around for all of us to gush and coo over the adorable footage. That felt normal; that felt good.

Later Neil and I went to bed around eleven and the restless night consumed us, tossing and turning in our bed. The warmth of Neil's body next to mine was no longer there when I reached out in the darkness. I got out of bed and searched for him with a desperate need for comfort. The clicking of his keyboard echoed through the hallway. He stood up from his desk and embraced me tightly, holding me until my eyes grew too heavy to stay open. I stumbled back to bed and fell into a deep sleep. When morning came, and the alarm blared, I hit snooze and allowed myself to drift back to sleep. The alarm rang for a second time. I knew I must face the inevitable. I couldn't run from cancer.

Moments after we picked our seats in the same empty and quiet waiting room, the nurse called my name. I chuckled at the strange sense of deja vu. She seemed almost robotic, moving through her routine. Maybe she saw ghosts sitting in the other empty chairs. My nerves were on edge, and my inappropriate laughter resulted from that nervous energy.

The doctor's confident stride down the hall to the exam room caught my attention. Neil and I waited anxiously. My stomach twisted in knots. I squeezed his hand tightly, seeking strength from his presence. The fear of what news she might deliver consumed me, but my biggest concern was how Neil would react. My heart ached for him as I prayed that whatever the doctor said wouldn't be too much for him to handle.

"I read the portal," I said before the doctor could get a word out edgewise.

"I wish they wouldn't post those reports on the portals until we've been able to talk to our patients," she said, her voice edged with frustration.

I clenched my jaw, fighting the urge to voice my dissent. I regretted not mustering the courage to confront my doctor about my decision to see the results before meeting with her. I wanted to inform her that being enlightened beforehand enabled me to process the situation and prepare myself rather than being caught off guard.

My cancer now had a name: Invasive Ductile Carcinoma. The doctor informed me the lump in my breast showed active cancer cells, but my lymph nodes were clear. I let out a sigh of relief. Still, she seemed concerned and added, "We won't have confirmation that the nodes are cancer-free until the surgeon removes and tests them."

I searched my mind for the courage to ask the million-dollar question. My voice quivered when I asked, "What stage of cancer am I facing?" The air around us felt thick and heavy, and I could feel the weight of my words hanging in the silence between us. The room seemed to hold its breath, waiting for the answer that would determine so much.

Her manicured nails traced the black-and-white lines on my lab report. "It's difficult to say definitively without surgery," she said gently. But from what we can tell, the tumor appears small."

The doctor scribbled an order for an MRI. Next, she asked me, "Which surgeon should I schedule your surgery with?"

My mind raced with uncertainty as I tried to make a decision that could potentially alter the course of my life. How could I determine the most skilled doctor for such a vital operation?

"I don't know," I said. The doctor offered to contact my primary care doctor to assemble a team. I felt too exhausted and unsure about researching surgeons and oncologists, so I took her up on her suggestion to let my primary care doctor decide.

When it was time for the MRI, the technician led me to the testing room. The cold metal and imposing size of the machine made my pulse quicken. I laid down, trying to remain still as instructed. The technician asked me what music I wanted to listen to. I blurted out, "Classic Rock!"

I quickly realized I made a terrible choice in music for a test where I needed to stay perfectly still. I changed my answer to soft jazz, hoping it would give me a sense of calm.

As the scan continued, my body began to protest. My knees ached from being bent awkwardly, my back screamed for relief, and my legs begged to be stretched. But I persevered, knowing any movement could skew the results. The discomfort grew, but I refused to give in to it. The stakes were too high to risk compromising the outcome.

When the test ended, I stretched my body like a cat on a windowsill waking up from a nap. After I put back on my bra and blouse, the nurse handed me a satchel filled with items. "With this bag, you're now a part of our cancer community," she said. "Feeling scared and angry is okay," she added compassionately.

I nodded, unsure what to say in return. I took the bag from her outstretched hand. "Sorry we couldn't give you better news today," she added. I forced myself to smile, eager to leave the room and breathe fresh air. Before I walked out the door, she called after me one more time. "Take care of yourself."

Neil's hands gripped the steering wheel, and I rummaged through the gift bag. I found a red throw and a brochure from Project 31. The blanket made me uneasy, as it reminded me of the cancer community in which my unwanted membership sent a sudden feeling of anger through me. I decided not to use it. Instead, I would wrap myself in the fuzzy gray blanket my son had given me as a gift for Christmas. As we passed a homeless person on the road, I immediately handed him the logoed blanket. It was better to keep someone else warm than to remind me of my battle with breast cancer.

The pamphlet in the bag gave me details about a group called Project 31. I knew I needed a support system – when my sister battled cancer, she told me research revealed females who attended breast cancer support groups had better odds of survival. She decided to join two clubs during her first year of breast cancer. My sister had always thought two was better than one. I was drawn to joining Project 31.

When we made it back home, I tidied myself up to go back to the office. I worried about how much salary I would lose due to this predicament. I wondered if I could keep myself afloat with a smaller paycheck. I burned through my vacation days when Neil and I went to Mexico for nine days a few months prior.

Some tips when having an MRI:
- Leave your jewelry at home.
- You can't wear magnetic lashes or magnetic eyeliner.
- Some hair extensions have metal clips, don't put them on the day of your MRI.
- Since you will be positioned on your stomach, don't eat a large meal before your MRI. You will be in this position for 15 to 25 minutes, and your breasts will be placed through two openings on the contoured MRI table.
- Drink large amounts of water 48 hours before your MRI to help the contrast dye flow.
- Drink large amounts of water after the MRI to help your body excrete the dye.
- If you think you might need an anti-anxiety medication, contact your referring doctor for a prescription to take the day of your MRI.

What to Expect:
- You will be asked to change clothing and put on the items they provide.
- Remove all metallic objects; don't forget about hairpins.

- If you have removable dentures, you will be instructed to take them out.
- You will receive an IV with contrasting dye.
- Even though earplugs and headphones are provided, the machine will still be very loud during scanning.
- You will enter the machine head first. Arm position may vary.

***

Internet Research:

Invasive Ductal Carcinoma (IDC) | Johns Hopkins Medicine

Invasive ductal carcinoma, also known as infiltrating ductal carcinoma or IDC, is the most common form of breast cancer, accounting for 80% of all breast cancer diagnoses.

Breast ducts are the passageways where milk from the milk glands (lobules) flows to the nipple.

Invasive ductal carcinoma is cancer (carcinoma) that happens when abnormal cells growing in the lining of the milk ducts change and invade breast tissue beyond the walls of the duct.

Once that happens, the cancer cells can spread. They can break into the lymph nodes or bloodstream, where they can travel to other organs and areas in the body, resulting in metastatic breast cancer.

***

Today's Quote:

"If it takes a village to raise a child, it takes a bloody army to battle cancer."

—Niyati Tamaskar

A Note to You:

My sweet friend, as you embark on this journey and plans start falling into place, I want you to take a moment to acknowledge your strength. You are in control. You have strength. Cancer doesn't. Rest, stay hydrated and well nourished. Keep fighting. Victory is within reach.

NOTES AND THOUGHTS

CHAPTER THREE

WANTING TO RUN

Cancer Post #5: Meeting the Surgeon: March 21st

I circled the dreaded Monday, March 21st, at 2:00 p.m. on my calendar with black ink. The date loomed over me like a storm cloud, waiting to rain down on my life. Every day felt like an eternity, awaiting the consultation. The cancerous tumor lingered inside my left breast. I feared it grew bigger every day, invading my body like an alien presence from a sci-fi horror movie. I wanted it out before it consumed me completely! But what if the cancer had already spread? These thoughts tormented me every moment.

I prepared myself for the appointment with my surgeon. I tried to distract my anxious thoughts by helping to organize a tea party for the residents where I worked. In the evenings, I concentrated on planning our wedding. We picked June 17th as our wedding day long before my cancer diagnosis. Despite my optimism, I wondered if Neil might not want to marry someone with breast cancer.

Neil and I planned to meet at the hospital's breast cancer center at two o'clock in the afternoon. I showed up early, walked to the elevator, and pushed the button. The doors opened, revealing a waiting room filled with women. Scanning the room, I saw women with bald heads, a gray pallor to their skin, and some with bloated bodies, while other forms were so thin, it looked like a gust of wind could knock them down. Faced with this sobering scene, an instinctual urge kicked in—I wanted to flee! I didn't belong here; I didn't want to end up as one of these unfortunate women.

Neil strode into the waiting room. His confident posture made him seem like a modern-day knight in shining armor. I felt a surge of relief as I watched him approach. He was my savior, my rock amidst the chaos of the hospital. His warm smile and kind eyes reassured me everything would be okay.

Later, as we sat in the small exam room, the surgeon pulled up images of the procedure on a screen, pointed out specific details, and explained her plan for a partial mastectomy and removal of two lymph nodes. Her calm and unhurried demeanor put us at ease. When she finished her presentation, she asked, "Do either of you have any questions?"

I blurted out, "When can we schedule the surgery, and how long will my recovery be?"

Her assistant checked the doctor's surgery schedule and set the date of March 31st. Surgery would take me away from work for an entire month. My mind raced with worry, and my chest felt like a bottle with too much built-up pressure. How could I possibly be away from work for so long? Conflicting thoughts ran through my mind.

Neil sensed my apprehension on our way to the parking lot. When we reached my car, he took my hand and said, "Don't worry about your lost wages. I'm happy to help with any of your bills. What I want you to do is focus on your recovery. I love you."

After Neil left, I sat in my car and tried to muster the motivation to return to work. But a gnawing feeling in my gut told me I needed more time. Time to process, grieve, and prepare for what was to come. My mind raced as I tried to figure out how to tell my grown children and close friends the news. With a deep breath, I picked up my planner and opened it. The pages were filled with appointments and reminders. I marked March 31st in black ink. The words "breast cancer surgery" stared back at me, stark and foreboding. A lump formed in my throat.

I dialed my wasbund, Horace. If you don't know what a wasbund is, it is your ex-husband. I think wasbund sounds nicer than ex. I needed his support in this difficult time, so I asked him to reach out to our children on my behalf. I explained the upcoming surgery and my recent cancer diagnosis. I wanted our children to process the news before I called them later that evening. Without hesitation, he offered his assistance and kind words that provided much-needed comfort.

I punched my sister Marcia's number into my phone. As soon as I shared the cancer news, I could hear the weight of her grief and despair. We had always been more than sisters, more like mothers to each other. Because our own mother had passed away from breast cancer, it was up to Marcia to take on the motherly role for me. There were many questions I longed to ask my mom, and I was remorseful for not comprehending what she endured during her treatments. I regret not being more empathetic towards her emotions. My sister and I reminisced when our mother showed us her mastectomy and said to us, "I feel like a freak. I look like Frankenstein."

My body became a battlefield, and I refused to surrender to this invisible enemy. I would fight with a relentless determination to defeat cancer, but I couldn't escape the constant fear gnawing at me. Would this disease ultimately claim my life?

***

Internet Research:

Lumpectomy (Partial Mastectomy): Purpose, Procedure, What to Expect (webmd.com)

Women who have this type of breast cancer surgery usually:

• Have a single tumor that's small – less than 4 centimeters in diameter.

• Have enough tissue so that removing surrounding tissue won't leave a misshapen breast.

• Are medically able to get surgery and follow-up radiation treatment.

***

Today's Quote:

"Once I overcame breast cancer, I wasn't afraid of anything anymore."

—Melissa Etheridge

A Note to You:

Amid our own struggles, we have the power to turn bad into good and help others along the way. Let's make it a point to remind our girlfriends to schedule their annual breast health checkups and encourage our guy friends to do regular self-exams. Some of the men might try to brush it off with a joke, but let's laugh with them and hope they'll remember our reminder the next time they're in the shower.

Cancer Post #6: Bone Scan: March 23rd

Anxiety followed me into my boss's office. I needed to discuss the time off required for the surgery. After taking a deep breath, I told her I would do my best to return to work within four to six weeks.

My boss, understanding and supportive, suggested I go to HR and apply for short-term disability. I forgot our company offered this benefit. Instantly, the weight of my worries lifted as I realized I wouldn't lose pay during my absence. As I filled out the paperwork for the application, a pleasant surprise greeted me - neither my health insurance nor 401K contributions would be deducted from the disability check. This was a huge relief, as I contributed significantly to my 401K. Without deductions, I would still receive my full salary while on leave. This positive news lifted my spirits and eased my mind about the upcoming surgery.

I filled out the Family and Medical Leave forms at a friend's suggestion. She told me that it would provide an added layer of protection, ensuring that I wouldn't be terminated or lose my healthcare benefits. Taking her advice to heart, I completed the necessary paperwork.

In the late afternoon, the Women's Breast Cancer Center called. My heart raced as I picked up the phone, dreading what they might reveal. They instructed me to come in for a baseline bone scan the following day. I struggled to keep up with the constant scheduling of appointments.

My life changed in an instant. One second, I was going about my routine, and then suddenly, everything was a chaotic blur.

The next day, while waiting for the bone scan, I was clueless about why somebody had ordered it. When I asked the tech aide, she told me I would need to ask my doctor. After the scan, I pulled up my medical records portal on my cell and scrutinized which doctor had requested the scans. Fortunately, all of them were at the same location, so I marched up to the oncologist's office and demanded to be informed why. I became angry and frustrated whenever I didn't have all the facts. A nurse soon entered the waiting room to explain they needed a baseline record of my bone density and to check if cancer had spread into my bones. This scan was necessary as treatments can cause thinning of our skeletal structure in some cases. I sighed deeply, feeling the weight of yet another worry added to my list.

I reflected on my job, working with senior citizens. I often overheard them say, "It feels like all I do is sit around in doctor's offices."

Now I understood what they meant, and I learned the necessity of checking my schedule every day to make sure I didn't miss any doctor's appointments.

***

Internet Research:

Family and Medical Leave (FMLA) | U.S. Department of Labor (dol.gov)

The Family and Medical Leave Act (FMLA) provides certain employees with up to 12 weeks of unpaid, job-protected leave per year. It also requires that their group health benefits be maintained during the leave. FMLA is designed to help employees balance their work and family responsibilities by allowing them to take reasonable unpaid leave for certain family and medical reasons. It also seeks to accommodate the legitimate interests of employers and promote equal employment opportunity for men and women.

***

Today's Quote:

"Every woman needs to know the facts. And the fact is, when it comes to breast cancer, every woman is at risk."

—Debbie Wasserman Schultz

A Note to You:

Take charge of your medical appointments. When a new appointment is scheduled, promptly note the date and time in your phone or planner. This proactive approach will help you avoid the stress of trying to remember everything. Missing an appointment or arriving late could result in a lengthy rescheduling process. Start your day by checking your calendar and patient portal to stay informed about any changes or additions. Be prepared for a busy schedule, as you will have multiple appointments to attend.

Cancer Post #7: YouTube: March 24th

As I counted down each of the next seven days until my operation, I constantly searched for new information. With every spare moment, I scrolled through Facebook, read books, watched YouTube, or listened to podcasts related to breast cancer. My obsession with learning more about the condition took over my life. YouTube, in particular, became my go-to source of knowledge; it was here I heard from various sources, including doctors, survivors, experts, and even mental health counselors. On YouTube, I discovered how to change my negative thoughts about cancer into positive ones. YouTube taught me about Invasive Ductile Carcinoma, the surgery, and the recovery process that lay ahead.

By the end of the week, I became cocky. I thought I knew more about breast cancer than the doctors on my team. Since I decided to control cancer rather than let it control me, I might as well instruct my doctors on how to do their jobs. I turned into a YouTube-educated prima donna. I figured I knew every holistic and traditional cancer treatment available.

As I absorbed information about breast cancer, I found comfort in knowing my early detection gave me a high survival rate. I felt empowered by the knowledge I acquired. Gratitude swelled within me for the selfless individuals who shared their experiences through videos and on private Facebook groups dedicated to cancer, as well as to the authors whose words of wisdom I could highlight in books, guiding me through this unfamiliar journey.

When I wasn't using the television to learn about my treatment options, I turned to entertainment to help numb my emotional ups and downs. After some time, I realized how many shows feature cancer as a plot line. Cancer is used in television shows to elicit an emotional reaction from viewers. Firefly Lane is a particularly gripping series featuring a character with cancer. If you are undergoing cancer treatment, be mindful of the stories you choose to watch – some could be more emotionally taxing than others.

My doctors may feel irritation when talking to me, considering how much I questioned them. Still, I refused to apologize for advocating for my health and survival. My well-being took precedence over any possible animosity they may have toward me.

I clung to every word of Dr. John P. Williams' YouTube videos about breast cancer. His series, Breast Cancer School for Patients, is a true gem. Dr. Williams breaks down the complexities of breast cancer in a simple and easy-to-understand way. I highly recommend these videos. You'll learn more than you ever thought possible!

My top picks of my favorite breast cancer Facebook groups. These groups have genuine and unfiltered emotions and insightful questions from fellow patients. The knowledge and information shared by other survivors is priceless.

Project 31 is a nonprofit group dedicated to the emotional restoration of breast cancer survivors and their families. I seriously don't know how I would have made it through breast cancer without this group.

Anastrozole, Letrozole, Exemestane, and Tamoxifen…Living with Side Effects. If your doctors recommend any of these drugs, and most likely they will, if you have estrogen-positive cancer, this site is valuable. Any of these hormone blockers are a tough pill to swallow, and you will need support.

Sex After Breast Cancer is the other group I needed. Sex After Breast Cancer is a private Facebook support group for women who experience physical and emotional pain in their intimate lives after undergoing treatment for breast cancer. Learn how to reclaim intimacy in your life through their contributing experts' guidance.

Breast Cancer Survivors Oklahoma is a non-profit organization that operates entirely through the service and commitment of its dedicated volunteers. They focus on being there for their members on a personal level, throughout their entire journey from the beginning, during and after breast cancer treatments are finished.

Check out Facebook to find Breast Cancer Support groups in your local area.

**

Internet Research:

https://www.cancercenter.com/community/blog/2020/10/questions-breast-cancer

If you or a loved one is diagnosed with breast cancer, one of the first things you can do is educate yourself about the disease. Open communication between patient and doctor is extremely important. And asking questions of your doctor may help you make more informed decisions about your breast cancer treatment.

**

Today's Quote:

"The period of greatest gain in knowledge and experience is the most difficult period in one's life."

—Dalai Lama

A Note to You:

Take a look at these recommended resources: books, YouTube channels, and Facebook support groups. They have been so helpful in my own journey with cancer. Don't be afraid to educate yourself about your diagnosis - knowledge is power. But remember, don't let the information scare you. Understanding what you're facing can give you the strength and courage to fight back.

Cancer Post #8: Symptoms: March 28th

My mind could not stop fixating on signs of cancer elsewhere in my body. My heart pounded as I thought about my monthly inspections of my breasts. Each time, my fingertips glided over each curve and angle, investigating for any sign of irregularity. But no matter how carefully I searched, I found nothing out of the ordinary:

- No lumps or bumps.
- No changes in shape or texture.
- No pain when I pressed around my breast tissue.

My thoughts kept returning to the extreme fatigue I would feel by the end of each day. Not having the energy to clean my house or go anywhere after work made me ask my co-workers if they were tired, too. Each one of them I asked said they were having an energy crisis. Since we were in the medical field, we decided it must be the aftereffects of Covid stress. We were essential workers and never got a day off at the height of the crisis. We figured the constant worry we would contract COVID-19 and maybe die or spread it to the elderly where we worked had taken its toll on us. At the time, that made perfect sense to me.

Worried about my dwindling energy, I turned to the authorities—my friends Linda and Luana. Naps and early bedtimes became a regular part of my routine. When I asked them for advice on how to combat this energy crisis, they thought of it as a side effect of our age. They suggested various vitamins and exercise, but I saw no improvement when I tried their suggestions.

***

Internet Research:

Early Cancer Warning Signs: Symptoms You Shouldn't Ignore | Johns Hopkins Medicine

This isn't fatigue similar to how you feel after a long day of work or play. Extreme fatigue that doesn't get better with rest can be an early sign of cancer. Cancer uses your body's nutrients to grow and advance, so those nutrients are no longer replenishing your body. This "nutrient theft" can make you feel extremely tired. There are lots of underlying causes of fatigue, many of them not cancer-related. If your symptoms are severe enough to affect your quality of life, call your doctor.

***

Today's Quote:

"Breathe, darling; this is just a chapter and not the end."

—S.C. Lourie

A Note to You:

The moment I heard the word "cancer," my world shattered. I ignored my body's cries for help for too long, and now I was paying the price. But you don't have to make the same mistake I did. Don't brush it off if you feel even a hint of exhaustion or lethargy. Go to your doctor immediately and demand to be tested for cancer. It could save your life.

Cancer Post #9: Surgery Day: March 31st

Before my surgery, I continued to work and found solace in interacting with patients and co-workers. When faced with the prospect of surgery, I realized how much I took for granted the routine of a typical workday. It was comforting to have a sense of normalcy in my life.

Throughout the week, Neil and I received kind offers from friends and family to keep him company during my surgery. I asked Neil, "Are you okay with not having anyone with you?"

With a look of surprise, he responded, "I'm not exactly a social butterfly like you."

"If you don't mind, would you please decline all the offers of help? I would feel like I would need to entertain them and put on a happy face. I'm scared. I don't have it in me to chit-chat with others."

Neil agreed and graciously turned down our friends and relative's offers of support.

The night before my surgery felt like a never-ending hourglass, each grain of sand representing the growing dread in my stomach. Neil and I sat on our front porch; our usual glass of wine replaced by a somber silence. The hummingbirds flitted around us, but their bright colors and playful chirps failed to cheer me up. I sipped on water from a wine glass. Neil's love for me radiated from his gentle touch, but even that couldn't ease the fear gnawing at me. What would he say when the bandages came off? Would he still see me as beautiful? A friend's words echoed in my head: "Don't ask the question if you're not ready for the answer."

But as much as I wanted to push those thoughts away, they lingered, casting a shadow over our relationship and future. Would we still be able to marry in June? Or would this surgery change everything?

The alarm blared at six a.m., and I immediately felt anxiety. Surgery was scheduled to start at two in the afternoon. Per standard procedure, I couldn't consume anything after midnight. As the morning wore on, my throat ached with dryness, and my stomach gnawed with hunger. I longed for a glass of water or a hot cup of coffee, but I knew it was forbidden. Denying myself of any liquid relief transpired into a temporary distraction from thinking about going under the knife.

The pre-surgery shower engulfed me in warm water, providing a false sense of security. But then the tears came, and they wouldn't stop. I wept as I scrubbed my left breast with the harsh anti-bacterial soap. "Why are you betraying me?" I cried.

My breast, the source of nourishment for my children, the symbol of my sexuality, and a defining aspect of my womanhood, remained silent. I half expected it to answer me, crazy, huh? I heard Neil calling from the hallway, "Who are you talking to?"

Feeling embarrassed, I shouted back, "Just singing in the shower."

As I towel-dried my skin, a paralyzing dread overcame me: no deodorant, no perfume, no body lotion—and, to make matters worse, not even a drop of makeup. Publicly exposing myself without my mask felt like a violation of everything I had worked so hard to create for myself. How could I possibly go out into the world like this? I never left the house without wearing my makeup. It felt as if I were being stripped of my dignity.

I put on my button-down shirt and sweatpants, as suggested in the pre-surgery paperwork. Heading into the garage and into the car, I felt uncomfortable and nervous, as if I were walking to the electric chair.

When we arrived at the hospital, we checked in with the admittance clerk. I felt the need to explain why I looked different without my false eyelashes. I could sense that she was indifferent and just doing her job.

We walked down the winding hallways to radiology, the first order of business: x-rays to confirm the position of the markers on my left breast. We waited at the glass window leading to the department, and the attendant gave me a buzzer that would signal my turn. Around us were scattered chairs and couches; we chose what looked like a comfortable sofa, but inspection revealed a revolting sight. The white leather was tattered, stained, and torn. My blood boiled as I seethed at the poor state of this supposed hospital furniture. How could they allow such filth? I stormed back to the window, demanding an explanation and expressing disgust. The uninterested girl rolled her eyes and advised me to report it on the survey following my surgery.

When I stepped into the surgery suite, my eyes took in the outdated and dilapidated state of the room. A large rip in the thin curtain caught my attention. I voiced my concerns to the nurse who came in to prepare me for the operation. Although I could sense Neil's annoyance with my complaints, my nerves were too high to keep silent. The nurse explained plans to renovate the room were on the agenda. The hospital postponed any non-essential upgrades due to COVID-19, which resulted in economic problems for the hospital, and they were waiting for the budget to return to healthy numbers.

The nurse started my IV, then looked at me and said, "I need to peek at your breast to mark it for the surgeon."

Laughter erupted from me, shaking my entire body. I went from agitated to hysterical in a matter of moments. I couldn't resist the urge to answer the nurse back with, "Peek-A-Boob," as she inspected my breast.

Neil and I played with our phones to kill time. A nurse and a man in scrubs came in and unlocked the brakes on the hospital bed, giving Neil and me a moment to kiss and say, "I love you."

The surgeon expertly performed a partial mastectomy and extracted two lymph nodes. As I emerged from the anesthesia, Neil awaited me in my small recovery room. The haze of medication made it difficult to stay lucid as I drifted in and out of consciousness. Despite the significant surgery, four hours later, I signed discharge papers and went home on the same day - just another outpatient procedure.

On our way home, Neil stopped at Braum's to get me a vanilla malt. That rich, creamy mix of milk and ice cream always brought me comfort.

When we got home, I took the pain pills and slept the rest of the evening.

***

Internet Research:

Lymph Node Removal (Lymphadenectomy) (cancercenter.com)

After a cancer diagnosis, the doctor may want to check the patient's lymph nodes for signs of disease. In a common procedure called a lymph node dissection, lymph node removal or lymphadenectomy, the surgeon removed one or more lymph nodes.

The lymph nodes are a part of the lymphatic system, also known as the lymphoid system. The lymphatic system is a network of lymph vessels, similar to a network of veins, found throughout the body. A clear fluid called lymph circulates through the vessels. Along the network are lymph nodes—small checkpoints that play important roles in the lymphatic system. Lymph nodes filter out germs, cancer cells, and foreign matter. They also house white blood cells called lymphocytes that fight infection.

Lymph nodes and the lymphatic system are essential to a person's general well-being, and because the body has hundreds of lymph nodes, it's generally safe to remove some of them.

***

Today's Quote:

"Breast cancer is scary and no one understands that like another woman who has gone through it too."

—Mindy Sterling

A Note to You:

My dear friend, I know you're scared about your upcoming surgery. I've been there. Your emotions will be all over the place, and anything and anyone can set you off. You need to warn whoever is going with you to be extra patient and understanding. And let's not even get started on the healthcare workers - they need to be on their toes, or else we'll bite their heads off. It's a shame we can't even stay overnight in the hospital anymore because of insurance companies. My wish for you is a smooth recovery.

Cancer Post #10: Recovery: April 5th

During my recovery, I spent most of my time dozing in bed or binging Netflix on the couch until exhaustion hit. Neil's sighs made me wonder if he perceived me as lazy, but he never vocalized it. My own guilt for not being productive plagued me and caused me to question his thoughts every time he entered the room.

The gauze dressing and bra corset they sent me home from the hospital in constricted my breath, making each inhale a struggle. The hospital gave me strict instructions not to remove the bandages or bra, even for something as simple as a shower for the next ten days. The thought of water seeping through the gauze and aggravating my condition filled me with dread. I could only stand under the shower with it hitting me from behind or on my right side. My breast remained shrouded in mystery, hidden under layers of thick wrappings. I wondered what horrors could be lurking beneath. At night, the tightness and constriction were almost unbearable. Desperate for relief, I relied on pain medication just to fall asleep. It made me think about how women must feel who strive for impossible beauty standards – like the nineteen-inch waist of the ladies in Gone with the Wind. When I complained, Neil reminded me, "It's only for ten days. You can do anything for ten days."

***

Internet Research:

Post-Lumpectomy Care Guide and Healing Steps (verywellhealth.com)

Proper post-lumpectomy care is vital for recovery and healing. Measures include keeping the wound clean, taking medication on a proper schedule, sleeping in the correct position, and more.

***

Today's Quote:

"It's our challenges and obstacles that give us layers of depth and make us interesting. Are they fun when they happen? No. But they are what make us unique. And that's what I know for sure… I think."

—Ellen Degeneres

A Note to You:

Always speak up about any pre-existing conditions or concerns before going into surgery. I have a friend who suffered from a hernia and worried that she would have trouble breathing and additional pain because of the tight corset pushing on her hernia. She spoke to her surgeon beforehand, and they made adjustments so it wouldn't aggravate her condition. Don't be afraid to advocate for your own comfort during recovery. It can make all the difference. Wishing you a smooth and comfortable recovery journey.

PEEK-A-BOOB

NOTES AND THOUGHTS

CHAPTER FOUR

CONFRONTING THE SHADOW

Cancer Post #11: FreedomBeckons: April 7th

In bed, my mind drifted between sleep and wakefulness. A nagging worry consumed me, impossible to shake. Uncertainty and stress weighed heavily, knowing it could contribute to a recurrence. It left me feeling powerless and reliant on Neil. But what if he couldn't handle seeing my scarred breast once the bandages were removed? I had no backup plan, no safety net.

I walked into his office and caught him engrossed in a baseball game on his computer. He warmly greeted me with a "Hello, sweetie." Uncertain of his availability, I inquired if, while he watched the game, he had a few minutes to talk. As most men do, he bristled at the phrase, "Can we talk?"

"No, go ahead," he said, turning down the volume.

"Our wedding is less than two months away..." My voice faltered, heavy with the unspoken pain and uncertainty of our future. "When you proposed, we never could have imagined cancer becoming a part of our lives. If you feel this is too much to handle, I wouldn't hold it against you for wanting to leave."

I watched as he stood up from his desk slowly and deliberately. His feet pounded the ground as he approached me, his expression unreadable. I could feel my stomach begin to churn as he stopped in front of me, planting his legs wide apart in a power stance. One hand firmly resting on his hip, and he raised his other hand, index finger towards me.

"Let's go get married right now! Put on your most beautiful dress and let's get to city hall. I love you so much, and nothing will ever change that."

His words filled my spirit with a wave of solace and calm. His unwavering assurance evaporated all my doubts and anxieties. I felt immense comfort in knowing our love would endure, no matter how much cancer had changed me. I felt a relieved grin slowly spread across my face.

I hugged him affectionately. "Thank you from the bottom of my heart. Let's stay with our June 17th plans so our family can witness our marriage." Never before had I experienced such unconditional love and support.

Life presents us with moments where we feel certain everything will be okay. This became that moment.

***

Internet Research:

Study Suggests Link Between Stress, Cancer Returning – NCI

For many cancer survivors, their worst nightmare is finding out that their cancer has come back. Even years after a seemingly successful treatment, cancer can start growing again, and scientists don't know how this happens.

Now, a new study suggests that stress hormones may wake up dormant cancer cells that remain in the body after treatment. In experiments in mice, a stress hormone triggered a chain reaction in immune cells that prompted dormant cancer cells to wake up and form tumors again.

But if you are stressed, that doesn't mean your cancer is going to come back, said the study's lead researcher, Michela Perego, Ph.D., of The Wistar Institute Cancer Center. Several intermediate steps need to occur, Dr. Perego said, at least according to their studies in mice.

"There could be many different ways to wake dormant cells. We've shown one mechanism, but I'm very confident this is not the only one," she added. The results of the new study were published in Science Translational Medicine.

While plenty of research has shown that stress can cause cancer to grow and spread in mice, studies haven't shown a clear link between stress and cancer outcomes in people. But it's difficult to study stress in people for several reasons, including challenges with defining and measuring stress.

Nevertheless, there could be many far-reaching effects of the new study findings, particularly in the realm of identifying new therapeutic leads, said Jeffrey Hildesheim, Ph.D., of NCI's Division of Cancer Biology, who was not involved in the research.

"This study is like a gateway that will likely open up numerous other research directions into the effects of cancer therapies and stress on dormant tumor cells," Dr. Hildesheim said. "It could also spark research into the effects of nerves and the nervous system on tumor growth," he said.

***

Today's Quote:

"Always remember that your present situation is not your final destination. The best is yet to come."

—Zig Zigler

A Note to You:

My dear friend, it's time to release the heavy burden that may be weighing on your mind. It's crucial for our well-being to confront our thoughts and fears head-on. We both understand the damaging effects of stress on our health, and our top priority now is to prevent cancer from returning. Don't be afraid to voice your concerns and put yourself first. Even if things don't go as planned, have faith that God and the universe will guide you towards what is meant for you. Take a leap of faith and let go of the stress before it causes further harm. Your health and happiness should come first.

Cancer Post #12: Unveiling the Hidden Truth: April 10th

On the tenth day after my surgery, anxiety coursed through me. It was finally time to remove the tight corset and dressing that had constrained my chest for what felt like an eternity. The thought of breathing freely again was like a dream come true. But at the same time, I feared seeing my chest exposed for the first time, dreading any possible disfigurement.

I asked Neil if he would stand by me as I unwrapped the mummy-like dressings. To ease the tension, as we stood in front of the mirror, ready to peel away the layers, he said, "You know I'm not a boob man. I like the girl next door look and a good brain. You have both," he said with a chuckle.

I cautiously inched each of the tiny hooks out of their eyelets. As I allowed the corset to slip from my body, I gasped in disbelief. The sudden absence of support was like a dream; my skin and chest felt so light and free! However, without the constriction, it felt like my chest wall had lost the ability to support itself.

I gently pulled layer after layer of the gauze dressing away from my body. My curiosity of what lie beneath now overruled my fear of what I might see. Before I unwrapped the final piece that still covered me, I looked at Neil. What I saw in his eyes was curiosity. It was like being back in high school Chemistry, waiting to see what would happen when you poured the final ingredient into the test tube.

I gasped when I saw the last piece of gauze fall, revealing the aftermath of my surgery. My breast was still intact, but there was a sunken area where the tumor had been removed. The scarring under my arm showed where the lymph nodes were taken out. When I tried to raise my left arm, I winced in pain. It was clear I needed to work on strengthening and stretching my left side.

Neil broke the silence, "You look great."

Joy flooded my heart when I embraced Neil, knowing he accepted me for exactly who I was. Standing by his side through sickness and health, all my insecurities disappeared.

My surgeon advised me on my recovery, instructing me to wear a front clasping sports bra at all times during the next few months. After finally getting rid of the suffocating corset, I eagerly put on my recently purchased green camouflage bra from Walmart. To my relief, it was incredibly comfortable. Still, I couldn't shake the instinctive urge to hold my left breast in place with my hand, fearing any movement would cause pain. I knew I needed to trust in my bra's support; otherwise, walking around holding my breast could draw unwanted attention in public spaces.

***

Today's Research:

Recovery From Breast Cancer Surgery (webmd.com)

Exercises After Surgery

Daily stretching exercises can help you regain mobility, but talk to your surgeon about when to start them.

Arm lifts. Sitting on the edge of a chair, or standing, lift both arms over your head with your elbows close to your ears. Hold for a count of five and repeat.

Arm swings. While standing, swing both arms forward and back from your shoulders (like a pendulum). Keep your elbows straight. Increase the distance of the swing each time. Repeat 10 times.

Wall climbing. Stand facing a wall with your feet close to the wall. Put your arms out in front of you with your hands on the wall. Climb the fingertips of both hands up the wall, until your arms are stretched over your head. Climb your fingers back down the wall.

***

Today's Quote:

"With the new day comes new strength and new thoughts."

—Eleanor Roosevelt

A Note to You:

I kept postponing the purchase of my boho wedding dress, unsure of what my body would look like. But now I knew. I started looking at dresses online. Those pictures of what might be my wedding dress gave me a flicker of excitement and hope. That's when I realized the importance of planning something that brings you joy during this challenging journey. It may seem trivial, but it can be a source of strength and positivity in the face of uncertainty. My advice to you, fellow pink sister, is to hold onto those moments of joy and let them guide you toward a more hopeful and optimistic outlook on this journey.

PEEK-A-BOOB

NOTES AND THOUGHTS

CHAPTER FIVE

GOD WINKS

Cancer Post #13: Divine Whispers: April 12th

During this cancer experience, I've doubted the Lord. I constantly questioned if I'd done something wrong or if He was punishing me. It's hard to understand why sickness exists and whether God truly cares about us. While many of my friends possess unwavering faith, I long for their certainty that everything is under God's control. However, numerous personality tests have labeled me a real-life Sherlock Holmes - constantly analyzing and asking endless questions, seeking answers to make sense of things.

    I rushed endlessly from one doctor's appointment to another, trying to make sense of my new normal. Surgeries and treatments consumed my life. Amid exhaustion, a strange presence often enveloped me, guiding me through the trials and tribulations. It felt like divine interventions were perfectly timed, offering hope in my darkest moments. These serendipitous occurrences could only be attributed to God's Winks.

    My first God Wink came from Janet. We had lost touch for years, but after my cancer diagnosis and before I shared it online, she messaged me on Facebook. She asked me not to think she was crazy, but God gave her a strong calling to pray for me and have her Bible study group do the same. When she sent me her message, only the doctors and my fiancé knew about my diagnosis. Janet spoke with strength and courage as she shared her divine mission despite her fears. I felt grateful for her obedience to the voice of God, and I felt connected with an even greater force watching over me - something spiritual, like a God Wink, assuring me that everything would be okay.

    One restless night, I sensed an urging from God. I texted Julie, a brave young woman battling rectal cancer who lost much of her physical dignity. Julie encouraged me to post my experiences about cancer on my Facebook page, just as she was doing. "God wants us as witnesses to bring hope and comfort to those in similar situations," she texted back. "You and I are vocal people. God needs us to witness and comfort others."

    Taking a deep breath, I obeyed Julie's suggestion and God's urgings to share my cancer experience on social media. I surrendered to His will. It felt like God was gently holding me in His arms, comforting me with assurance He was guiding me down this path. Another God Wink.

In the middle of dealing with cancer, I learned the eye complications from my failed cataract surgery one year earlier still lingered. Insurmountable anger welled inside me—a fury so deep it reached my core and rattled my faith. "God, how can you do this to me? I'm already managing cancer—do I really have to tackle this, too?"

As we gathered for our morning huddle at work, Chaplain Adrian cleared his throat and asked if he could pray for me. I felt a heavy sense of apprehension in the air. His eyes searched mine, almost as if already knowing my answer. Bleakly, I nodded, feeling the weight of my doubt and saying, "Yes, but it won't make a difference."

He closed his eyes in prayer, and I couldn't help but feel skeptical. But then, something strange happened. A sense of calm filled the room, and I listened intently as he begged for inner peace and healing on my behalf. The next day, as I battled through the pain and confusion of my cancer diagnosis, that same peace surrounded me like a protective cocoon. Friends appeared at just the right moments, offering prayers and gentle encouragement along my journey. Each interaction felt like an intervention, a personal God Wink from above.

My beloved sister Willow was always there to remind me of the spiritual power of the universe. Whenever I felt lost or in need of guidance, she arrived with something I didn't even know I needed—a physical gift like incense or a note that spoke directly to my current struggles. Her deeply held beliefs in the power of love and connectedness were so strong they manifested themselves in the physical world. For me, they proved more God Winks. For her, they were from the universe.

My family is an incredible source of strength and stability. One day, I opened my front door to greet my eighteen-year-old grandson. He stepped inside and tightly hugged me. His sweet embrace cloaked me with God's Winks.

When my fingers intertwined with my fiancé's, I melted into his comforting presence. Neil listened to me without passing judgment, offering a sanctuary to release all of my joys and sorrows. During these moments, I felt as if God himself winked at me, reaffirming that this was exactly where I belonged.

One day while clicking through my Audible app, looking for a good fiction or murder mystery to download, something stirred inside me. God reached out His hand and placed it gently on my shoulder. I stopped searching for fiction and felt drawn toward more spiritually fulfilling selections. The power of that moment brought clarity and understanding to the situation; it felt like a big wink from Heaven telling me, "Trust in Me, and I will guide you where you need to go."

Immediately, this book popped up on my screen: The Cry of the Soul: How Our Emotions Reveal Our Deepest Questions About God. This book explores what Scripture says about our darker emotions and points us to ways of honoring God as we faithfully embrace the full range of our emotional lives.

The next day, while walking through the halls of my workplace, a gentle hand touched my shoulder. I turned to find Nettie, an older woman with kind eyes and a soothing voice. She smiled at me warmly and said she read my Facebook posts about cancer. She confirmed to me sharing my story as I lived it proved helpful to others. Yet another of God's infinite winks.

I'm thankful for the overwhelming love and support from family, friends, and strangers. Their comforting words and embraces, whether in-person or virtual, provided a source of strength for me. Despite the challenges of my journey, I felt a gentle nudge from God every day, reminding me to remain hopeful. I know the internal storms of hormones and emotional ups and downs can be difficult to navigate, but I asked for the grace to be kind to myself when surrounded by darkness. Keep sending the winks, dear Lord – for they are indeed blessings I am grateful for.

***

Internet Research:

Spiritual Support When You Have Cancer | Cancer.Net

Living with cancer can feel like living with uncertainty. Sometimes that uncertainty can lead you to think about questions in the context of your personal spirituality. You may have been a spiritual or religious person before you had cancer or it may be something you did not think about before.

Spiritual support can help you identify sources of strength and strategies for coping. Finding ways to cope with and process your experience is an important part of your overall cancer care. Many patients, and their loved ones, report that spiritual support and care helped them during cancer.

***

Today's Quote:

"God, Winks are better than coffee and chocolate!"

—Shelley Stutchman, Author of *PEEK-A-BOOB* and Breast Cancer Survivor

A Note to You:

As you journey through this book, my dear pink sister, know that I have fought countless spiritual battles. And if you struggle with your faith, give yourself some mercy. You are facing many challenges, and healing goes beyond just the physical. May you be blessed with countless God Winks along the way.

NOTES AND THOUGHTS

Chapter Six

MY TUMOR'S ADVENTURE

Cancer Post #14: The BRCA Gene Test: April 18th

My oncologist ordered the BRCA gene test. On one hand, I wanted to know whether or not I carried this cancer gene, knowing it could potentially affect my daughter and granddaughters. On the other hand, the thought of passing down an inherited mutation for generations filled me with guilt. My stomach twisted into a sickening knot. If the test proved I had this gene, I vowed to beg forgiveness from my family. Somehow, I felt responsible for their potential misfortunes.

    I didn't feel peace as I waited for the test results. It seemed inevitable it would confirm my fears - I carried the gene responsible for breast cancer. The fact my mother, sister, and I all battled the disease only added to my unease. To top off the worry, Horace (our daughter's father and grandfather to our granddaughters) held a family history of cancer - his mother died of colon cancer, his sister succumbed to breast cancer at just thirty-nine, and his brother lost his battle with lung cancer before even reaching fifty. The weight of this knowledge left me feeling powerless.

    One month later, I received the test results, negative for the gene. A wave of relief washed over me, knowing I was not passing this disease down to my daughter and granddaughters.

    In the near future, our daughter will undergo genetic testing to determine whether this gene has been passed down from her father's side. I fervently hope she is clear of this inherited mutation.

***

Internet Research:

Breast Cancer: Ask Health Professionals (msn.com)

BRCA gene testing is a type of genetic testing that looks for specific mutations in the BRCA1 and BRCA2 genes. These genes are essential for maintaining the stability of a cell's genetic material because, when they are in good working order, they generate proteins that aid in the repair of damaged DNA. However, mutations in these genes can result in a markedly higher chance of acquiring several malignancies, most notably ovarian and breast cancer. The test is frequently advised for those with a family history of these malignancies since it might offer essential risk assessment and management information. Although a positive test does not ensure the development of cancer, it does signal an increased risk, which can inform decisions about early detection and preventative tactics. It is important to note that BRCA mutations account for a small percentage of all breast and ovarian cancers.

***

Today's Quote:

"We have two options, medically and emotionally: give up or fight like hell."

—Lance Armstrong

A Note to You:

As women, we tend to blame ourselves for everything. It's like society has ingrained it into our minds. But here's the thing: We can't let that fear of knowing stop us from taking the test. There's power in knowing and taking control of our health and the health of future generations. Rather than feeling guilty, we should treat ourselves to something yummy and enjoy every bite of it guilt-free.

Cancer Post #15: Tale of My Vacationing Tumor: April 21st

My cell phone rang, startling me from my train of thought. The Breast Cancer Center's number showed on my screen. My gut tightened. I pressed the answer button, bracing myself for my oncologist's voice on the other end. After my surgery on March 31st, my tumor was sent to a lab in California for testing. I pictured the blob lounging on a sunny beach while waiting for its results. This test determined if I needed chemotherapy or not - the moment of truth. If my score was 25 or below, no chemo; if it was 26 or higher, chemo was inevitable. I crossed my fingers and awaited my doctor's verdict...24! A joyous "Yabba Dabba Do" escaped my lips. But as the good news sunk in, so did a twinge of worry - my score loomed dangerously close to the threshold. My oncologist mentioned insurance coverage and how it could affect decisions on whether or not to proceed with chemo. It amazed and terrified me how much our fate can depend on arbitrary numbers and percentages, as well as insurance coverage. However, I did a little happy dance when I hung up the phone.

***

Internet Research:

The Oncotype® DX Breast Recurrence Score | OncoLink

Oncotype Dx® is a genomic laboratory test that helps guide treatment decisions for people with early-stage invasive breast cancers. Genomic tests look at the genes in tumors. This can tell us more about your risk of the cancer coming back. Genomic tests are not the same as genetic tests. Genetic tests look for a single-gene mutation in your body (like BRCA 1 and 2). Genomic tests look at the genes in the tumor.

After you have surgery (lumpectomy or mastectomy), pieces of the tumor are sent to Exact Sciences Laboratory where the test is done. It will take about 2 weeks for your provider to get the results. Scientists look at the tumor samples. They measure the amount of 21 specific genes in the tumor tissue. Sixteen of the genes are cancer-related; the other 5 are used as "reference" genes. Based on the amount of each of these genes, a score is assigned. This is called the Recurrence Score (RS). This score is on a scale of 0-100. Higher scores mean there is a greater risk of recurrence (cancer coming back). A higher score also means you are likely to benefit from getting chemotherapy to reduce the risk of recurrence. Your recurrence score, in combination with your age and the size and grade of your tumor, will help pick the best treatment for you to prevent a recurrence.

How the score is used for treatment decisions depends on your menopausal status and if you had cancer in your lymph nodes.

A postmenopausal person with or without cancer in the lymph nodes (positive or negative nodes):

A score of 0-25 indicates a low risk of recurrence. Adding chemotherapy to your treatment will not add any benefit. The risks of chemotherapy would outweigh the benefits of having chemotherapy.

- A score of 26-100 indicates a high risk of recurrence. The benefits of chemotherapy in preventing a future recurrence outweigh the risks.

A premenopausal person with no cancer found in the lymph nodes (node-negative):

A score of 0-15 indicates a low risk of recurrence. Likely the risks of chemotherapy would outweigh the benefits of having chemotherapy.

A score of 16-25 indicates a low to medium risk of recurrence. There may be a small benefit to adding chemotherapy to your treatment. You may get the same benefit by taking medicines to stop your ovaries from making estrogen along with hormone therapy. Your oncology team will talk about the risks and benefits with you.

- A score of 26-100 indicates a high risk of recurrence. The benefits of chemotherapy are greater than the risks of side effects.

***

Today's Quote:

"Do not partner with fear to help you make decisions."

—Jeannette Gregory

A Note to You:

I've talked to many women who have yet to learn their Oncotype score or if they even had the test. It's crazy, right? This number can be life-changing, yet some doctors don't even bring it up. If your oncologist has yet to mention it, make sure you ask. If they didn't order this test for your tumor, find out why. You may be tired from surgery, but you have to keep fighting for your life and advocating for yourself.

Cancer Post #16: Chemotherapy: April 23rd

I feel incredibly fortunate that I didn't have to undergo chemotherapy. However, I know that many of you reading this book may have to go through the experience. My sister was kind enough to share her own journey with chemotherapy years ago. Despite its difficulty, she is still alive today thanks to the treatment. My sister's story...

***

"My doctor told me I had a suspicious lump, but the mammogram didn't show it. The same thing happened for three more years. Then, after the fourth year, I was sure I had breast cancer. I could feel that lump slowly growing larger, but the mammograms were always clear. I worried that making an appointment just two months after another good result would label me as a hypochondriac, and anything I said about my health would be ignored. I had to take action, but I didn't know what to do other than talk to my doctor about it, even if he didn't believe me. My worry was for nothing, and the doctor authorized another mammogram. Instead of relaxing, I was terrified that it wouldn't show anything again and I would die untreated.

The fifth time, they found the cancer with the help of the radiology technologist. She was a friend, and because of that, she took time to pinpoint it on the image with a marker so it couldn't be missed, and it wasn't. That same day, I had several more tests and another visit with my doctor, who made an appointment with an oncologist for me. Instead of fear and uncertainty, I finally felt relief. I was going to get help.

I was prepared for any treatment I needed, and I even had a plan. I was going to live as normally as I could and work through any pain or discomfort that came with the treatment. My life wasn't going to change, and I would never give in to the discomfort of the cure for my cancer. I was oblivious to what chemo would do.

I had a mastectomy and lymph nodes removed, then a port installed under my skin for the needle that would deliver the chemo solution. Just two weeks after the diagnosis, I was sitting in a waiting room for my first chemo treatment. I told Shelley I could go alone, but she insisted on accompanying me. Thank goodness for my caring sister because reality hit as I looked around the room and noticed women with scarves or turbans on their heads to hide baldness and men with only wisps of hair left on their heads. They looked sick. Some pretended to have a jolly demeanor and joked with the staff, while others looked quietly defeated, and then my hands started to shake. Without saying a word, Shelley took my hand and gently held it in both of hers, and we waited for my name to be called.

The treatment area was decorated in soft earth tones and paintings of beautiful landscapes on the walls. The room was lined with rows of brown reclining chairs that I knew were comfortable because I worked in a furniture store and had sold them to the doctor just a few months earlier. There had to be some kind of irony in that.

Shelley and I were both impressed with the kindness of the staff as they went through the routine of getting me ready for my first of six treatments. I was starting to relax and tons of questions came to mind. The big question was, what is this stuff they are putting in my body going to do to and for me?

To say it bluntly, chemotherapy is a poison designed to kill cancer cells and other types of cells. Thankfully, the nurse didn't use such straightforward language when answering my question. However, her response did little to ease my worries.

Chemo is not just one drug but a mixture that is used to target different kinds and stages of cancer. Chemotherapy drugs can't distinguish between healthy cells and cancer cells. That is the reason for the many side effects that are experienced during treatment. The healthy cells are able to rebound while the cancer cells die.

I am a balance between an optimistic and pessimistic person, but at that time, the only thing that came to mind was that I was watching poison dripping into my body. I needed the courage that my optimistic side would bring, so I decided to imitate the jolly people that I had seen in the waiting room. As soon as the nurse left, I whispered to Shelley that I felt more nervous than a student waiting to be scolded by the principal and possibly have my misbehavior put on my permanent record, which was rumored to ruin our chances of having a good job when we grew up.

That was the hint that Shelley needed to help me get through that first treatment. She reminisced about all the times we got in trouble growing up. We laughed so hard that the other people looked our way with approval. The hours flew after that, and the time came to remove the drip, only to replace it with another one that I was to wear home and come back the next day to have it removed. That was something I hadn't expected. I wore the deep blue bag wrapped around my waist that held the additional chemo. The fluid that was dripping into my body was saving my life, not ending it, but I felt no elation at that thought. Wasn't it just a few weeks earlier that I was afraid I would not be treated? The treatment was happening, and no matter how bad I felt, I needed to focus on the future when I would be healthy again.

As my first chemo evening at home progressed, I slowly developed the worst headache I ever had. My husband, Larry, thought I should call my doctor or go straight to the ER. Not thinking very clearly, I refused because I was sure nothing could be done about side effects.

The next day, my oncologist told me that a lot could be done to help make me more comfortable. To ignore issues caused by the chemo was damaging to my health. I was dehydrated, and the pain had done me no good. His scolding was kind, but I had to work hard to keep from crying. That was when I found out cancer, and especially breast cancer, was often the cause of depression. I was given an infusion for dehydration and the headache, as well as medicine for depression. Before I left, my oncologist gave me a warning that I took as a joke I didn't quite get. He told me not to eat much of my favorite foods because after the treatments were over, I would no longer like those foods.

I went home with two weeks to recover. The time after that first chemo treatment was out of control. My head started to itch so strongly that it was almost unbearable. There was relief in tugging on my hair, but when I did that, it came out in handfuls. When I didn't, it fell out anyway. Leaving clumps of hair everywhere, I put my head. The hair that was falling all over the house seemed disgusting to me, and even though it was August, I started to wear a knitted hat to contain the mess my hair made.

The loss of my hair was a fair exchange for my life, but I had a lot to learn. My eyelashes and eyebrows eventually came out, and then I had no hair on my body at all. Even the hair in my nose came out, which was a very strange feeling and gave my voice a nasal tone.

The first week after each treatment, I didn't want to eat at all, and when I did, I felt nauseous. Then I started to get better and with that ravenous. My husband was so relieved to see me eating again that he took me to my favorite restaurant where I could get delicious crab legs, and I ate and ate. I couldn't stop eating even when I didn't want food.

I found a support group through the hospital and an online support chat group. Those two groups were my anchor that kept me on track to recovery. They were a wealth of information that was even more advanced than what I received from the professionals, and they helped me make good decisions about my health. I also learned that compulsive eating was common, and both groups complained about gaining weight. I thought it was totally unfair that I got the only kind of cancer that caused a person to gain weight.

Even though I tried, I couldn't live as I had before the treatment because my body wouldn't let me. Keeping my job was out of the question, but I found at-home work that I could do as I was able and provided the money I had been contributing to the family budget. After several more treatments, even that became too much. I had taken out an insurance policy just for cancer that was paid directly to me. It solved financial problems but not the sinking feeling that I was no longer a useful person, I had become someone who contributed nothing. My oncologist gave me stronger antidepressants that didn't appear to do any good. After a few weeks, I was pushing myself to smile and create a stronger will that wasn't truly there.

The people in my support groups became my dear friends, and we were always there for one another. During that time, they encouraged me and gently pushed me to fight the depression I was feeling. They were the relief that pills couldn't provide.

We were fighting for our lives together, and we were stronger together. No one in my face-to-face group had been diagnosed early, and some of us had been diagnosed very late.

Every good day was Christmas morning, and every bad day brought gratitude that we were still breathing. Living so close to the edge turned every one of us into a drama queen. We laughed hard and cried deeply.

The hospital provided us with a meeting room on the main floor but moved us upstairs with blinds on the windows that we were instructed to leave closed. The reason caused all twelve of us to break into rolling on the floor type belly laughs. When new ladies joined our group, their first concern was how they would look after their mastectomy or lumpectomy. Some of us would take off our blouses to show how our chests looked right after the surgery, and others to show the appearance of different kinds of reconstruction. When we met on the first floor, unknown to us, we could be seen and were seen by high school boys who peeked around the bushes that we thought were hiding the windows. Oops.

A young woman with beautiful red hair joined our group. She was very soft-spoken, but when surrounded by caring women, she felt comfortable enough to tell her story. She had just been diagnosed and was upset about losing her hair. Her husband, a local minister, thought it wouldn't reflect well on him if she showed vanity about her hair. His cold behavior broke her heart.

She was desperate to talk to someone who cared and wanted to join our group, but her husband refused to allow her to join us because he heard a rumor that we stood naked in front of a window. Oh my, how rumors spread.

She attended our group when she could, she snuck away to our meetings and we did what we could to encourage her and give her hope. She had planned to leave her husband and move out, but her breast cancer escalated, which made leaving him no longer an option. She only lived a couple of months more, but she was one of us, and we shed many tears the night we were told of her passing. In sympathy for her, we all wore pink to her funeral.

Her time with us didn't ease her into death but gave her friends who cared for her for the short time she had left.

The loss of one of our group felt very personal. Our meetings were often full of laughter and taking advantage of the refreshments the hospital provided. Now, with the first death of one of our own, our meeting room echoed with the kind of whisper in our voices that was usually only heard during solemn occasions as we talked about our own mortality. The refreshments remained untouched. We had no jokes to tell. No family stories to share or complaints about trivial problems. We knew that not all of us would beat the enemy in our bodies. The room must have looked like normal women having a meeting in casual clothes, but we knew we were soldiers battling with our own bodies. The comfort we gave one another that night was a lifeline of hope. Others were lost, but even more were recovering. That was the hope we clung on to.

When I finished my chemo treatments, I received advice from those who had already passed it, and I gave advice to the new members.

A couple of weeks later, my radiation treatments started. I expected radiation to be a breeze compared to chemo. I wouldn't even need anyone to drive me to the daily appointments. My first visit was to have the area of my body that would be targeted by the radiation machine carefully measured and marked. This took over an hour and was done in a freezing cold, medically spooky room. I had been spoiled by staff that was considerate, kind and there for my every need.

The woman who did the measuring matched the room. But she certainly wasn't silent and immediately started sharing her ideas on a controversial issue. Her beliefs were the opposite of mine, and as she spoke, she was marking my body to be radiated. I remained quiet because I was concerned about the possibility that I might irritate her and she would mark a spot over my heart or some other vulnerable organ.

The actual radiation treatments lasted only minutes and people more tactful than the first lady operated the machine. Since I saw the staff every day for seventy-five working days, we became friendly, and I took their advice to heart. I was not to wear a bra, and I was to rub an ointment on my chest several times a day to ease the burns the radiation would cause. I followed their advice, and my burns were minimal, no worse than a bad sunburn. The technicians shared bits of hospital gossip with me and told their own stories of encounters with the same lady who didn't impress me. They felt more like friends than personal. The treatments were not painful. That came later. Every day, I felt weaker than the day before and needed an enormous amount of sleep. In some ways, it disrupted my life more than the chemo. I was so tired that I couldn't even go to my support meetings. The ladies noticed that I hadn't been going and regularly visited or called. My hair was growing back and I was anxious to stop wearing a wig. I had missed the feeling of wind blowing my hair and I was so ready to have it again. I vowed never to cut it again. That was a vow that I broke since I am not good at hair styling and not happy with stringy hair. Finally, on a windy Valentine's Day, I had my last treatment. The staff surprised me with a cake and some small gifts. I left for home cured.

I thought it was over and no one told me differently. The worst was yet to come, but those first days were for celebrating. My husband and I enjoyed the relief that I was well until I stopped enjoying it. I would stare blankly at the TV and had no desire to do anything. I blamed myself for being so gloomy and tried to force myself to happy up. It didn't work. I was becoming obsessed with thoughts of the cancer returning. I blamed myself for not appreciating being a survivor.

I had refused to take chemo in pill form as a preventive measure after researching the side effects and listening to my support group. Most of them also refused it or quit taking the pills after trying them for a month or two. Maybe I made a mistake in not taking the pills. No medicine, no little soldiers in my body keeping the cancer cells away. With every cough, freckle, or little bump, I imagined it had returned, and depression became a way of life. My husband didn't understand what was going on, and I was irritated with myself because I couldn't let it go.

I hadn't been attending my support group, but I decided to go back. Thank goodness I did. I guess fate stepped in because, on that first time back, our speaker talked about post-treatment depression, which is especially common in breast cancer survivors. It wasn't some fault in me but common.

I listened to the other survivors' stories of depression and felt less alone. My oncologist gave me a stronger antidepressant. I was getting help and working hard to appreciate my life again. Emotional recovery from breast cancer takes years, but it gradually gets better, and life becomes good again.

If I never had breast cancer, I would never have met the ladies in my support groups who became dear friends. I knew what to do to help my sister when she was diagnosed with breast cancer. It was a long journey, but I survived better than before. I have the gift of life and I know how to take advantage of that gift.

I regret not listening to my doctor, who warned me not to eat my favorite foods. He was right. I didn't like crab legs anymore."

***

Internet Research:

Chemotherapy for breast cancer - Mayo Clinic

Chemotherapy for breast cancer uses drugs to target and destroy breast cancer cells. These drugs are usually injected directly into a vein through a needle or taken by mouth as pills.

Chemotherapy for breast cancer frequently is used in addition to other treatments, such as surgery, radiation or hormone therapy. Chemotherapy can be used to increase the chance of a cure, decrease the risk of the cancer returning, alleviate symptoms from the cancer or help people with cancer live longer with a better quality of life.

***

Today's Quote:

"Before I started chemotherapy treatments, I wrote down the best advice from doctors, family, friends, books, and survivors and created an 'Owner's Manual' to help me take care of myself. It would remind me that cancer is doable."

—Regina Brett

A Note to You:

My soul sisters and brothers who have undergone chemotherapy speak of the harshness and challenges of the treatment. But now, it's like a distant dream, and they are grateful to be alive and thriving. I may not have personally experienced chemo, but I know that it brings healing to so many and restores the light in their lives. To those embarking on this journey, know that my daily vibes of love and healing are with you always. Peace and blessings, my friends.

NOTES AND THOUGHTS

# CHAPTER SEVEN

CORDING AND LYMPHEDEMA

Cancer Post #17: Hidden Hazards: April 30th

Saturday night, around ten p.m., I couldn't ignore the tightness in my left arm any longer. Since Friday, my arm had not felt quite right, so I brushed it off as a minor issue. A lump started to form on the inside of my elbow. It seemed to grow before my eyes, resembling half a golf ball beneath my skin. Panic set in. Fearful it could be something serious, a sense of dread washed over me.

I searched extensively on YouTube and the Internet to find some answers. While researching my symptoms, all the information I gathered suggested I might have lymphedema or cording. Why didn't any of the doctors tell me lymphedema and cording might happen weeks or months after the operation after lymph node removal? What other surprises could happen to my body?

My arm throbbed, and the growing lump in my elbow felt tender to the touch. Anxious thoughts raced through my mind as I noticed my left breast swelling at the same time. Desperate for help, I shared a photo of the lump on my Project 31 Facebook page. I received an immediate flood of comments. Countless suggestions and tips poured in from members who were well-informed about lymphedema and cording. Someone mentioned calling the 24/7 phone number for the Breast Cancer Clinic and provided me with the number. I found comfort among my fellow P31 members. With their support, I no longer felt panicked and could take action to move forward.

I grabbed my phone and punched in the on-call number. After navigating through a list of options for my specific issue, I received a callback fifteen minutes later. The voice on the other end belonged to a nurse practitioner, who listened intently as I described my worries and symptoms. She didn't judge me or make me feel stupid; instead, she calmly walked me through each detail. "Is the swelling warm? Do you have a fever?" she probed, her tone full of concern and professionalism.

"No, and no," I answered.

She assured me it was OK to wait until Monday to call my doctor unless those symptoms she asked about occurred or any other warning signs presented themselves. Thankfully, none did.

On Monday, I took charge of my health and contacted my doctor to add another appointment to my jam-packed calendar. Through my research, I knew that if I acted quickly on the signs of cording or lymphedema, I could optimize my chances for successful treatment.

***

Internet Research:

CONDENSED_Lymphedema_ASelfCareGuide.pdf (unclineberger.org)

Lymphedema is a buildup of fluid in the skin of an arm or leg or in your chest, breast, head or neck. Normally, your body carries a clear fluid called "lymph" through a special network of vessels and nodes. This network is called your lymphatic system. Lymphedema happens when damage occurs to this system and lymph cannot move through the body. This can happen after cancer treatments, including surgery and radiation. If the lymph fluid cannot be moved through your body, it can cause swelling in that area.

***

Today's Quote:

"Cancer may have started the fight, but I will finish it."

—Unknown

A Note to You:

I want to give you a crucial piece of advice. When I needed the on-call number for emergencies, I didn't have it. I don't know if it was given to me in my initial paperwork. If you received a hot-line number, jot it down, keep it visible, and put it in your cell phone. You never know when you may need it in a critical situation. Unfortunately, I learned this the hard way. Don't make the same mistake I did, "live and learn," as they say. Ensure your partner or caregiver knows the number, so that person can help in an emergency. It will save you a lot of unnecessary stress.

Side note: In my ongoing research about cancer, I learned there are over 200 different types of cancer, which is why there will never be a singular "cure" for cancer.

Cancer Post #18: Mysterious Disappearance of Symptoms: May 2nd

My tension eased as the oncologist's office nurse swiftly arranged an appointment for the same day. It lifted a heavy burden off my shoulders, knowing I wouldn't have to endure days or even weeks of waiting to see a specialist. At precisely 1 PM, I sat across from Diane, grateful for the chance to receive treatment from her dedicated center for Lymphedema and Cording.

As she examined me, I felt the swelling in my elbow dissipate, almost as if it was never there. The heavyweight in my left breast disappeared. It wasn't the first time this had happened - whenever I needed medical help, my pain seemed to miraculously vanish. Was it a mere coincidence, or the collective power of all the prayers and well-wishes from my loved ones finally working its magic?

Cutting Diane off before finishing her sentence, I declared with superiority, "According to what I've read, I have cording and maybe lymphedema."

Diane didn't seem rattled or offended. She explained cording is a side effect of having lymph nodes removed because of breast cancer. A cord, or web of cords, develops under the skin on the inside of your arm. This rope-like tissue can be uncomfortable and make it difficult to use your arm normally, but there are treatments that can help. She told me Lymphedema occurs when the lymphatic fluid does not adequately drain from the limb region because of the damage to the lymph nodes. It can be characterized by mild to severe swelling in the limbs. There is no cure for lymphedema. Treatments aim at reducing swelling and controlling the pain.

As I listened to Diane's words, conflicting emotions and questions flooded me. No cure? I would have it for the rest of my life? Did I hear her right? This news didn't fit into my plans. In just two months, I planned to walk down the aisle, and now this cruel side effect could still disrupt my plans for "happily ever after."

Diane broke the silence, "I need to measure your arms and do some range of motion tests. I'll also perform manual palpations on your arms, breast, underarm, and back. Then I can determine if it is lymphedema, cording, or both."

She moved quickly, measuring each arm precisely before proceeding to the range-of-motion tests. Gently, she started manual palpations on my arms, breasts, underarms, and back, probing deeply into my skin, holding my fate in their grasp.

After the physical probing, she tapped away on her computer, saying she needed to run some calculations. She turned to me with an expression of understanding and softly said, "I have found two issues. You have cording in your arm, lymphedema in your arm and hand, and swelling in your left breast."

My spirits plummeted. For a brief moment, I could not see how I could conquer both lymphedema and cancer at the same time. Diane's measured yet gentle voice calmed me as she established a plan of action. "Weekly visits until August, then we'll reassess," she said. "You will also need to wear a compression sleeve."

I gazed at the ceiling tiles while she searched for a catalog of compression sleeves. Memories of when my sister wore hers swirled in my mind. They were not attractive. One of my sister's managers told her not to wear the sleeve at work because it didn't fit the culture of the department. I asked, "How long do I have to wear it?"

Diane answered, "You can take it off at night when you sleep."

"What I'm asking is, will I be done with it after August?"

As her eyes met mine, I could see a deep understanding of the gravity of my situation in them. "This is a lifelong condition," she sighed.

Her words hung heavy, sinking into my skin like lead. I tried to comprehend what this meant for me – for my life, my dreams, and my future. The weight of it all felt suffocating. How would my body respond? What changes would I need to make? What sacrifices would I have to endure? I knew there were no easy answers.

Diane handed me the catalog. I looked inside, and a dazzling array of compression sleeves popped from the pages. They looked stylish and sleek, worlds away from the bulky sleeves my sister used to wear. An intense determination flared within me; I wouldn't be beaten by this. Instead of feeling sorry for myself, I'd pick one of these designer-looking sleeves and flaunt it with pride. I would be a trendsetter in the outside world. Yes, everyone would want one if I rocked it with a badass attitude. With a smirk, I showed her which sleeves to order.

I selected a beige skin-colored sleeve for work, determined to maintain the company's strict dress code. But I knew I needed to shake things up in my off-hours, so I picked the wild tattoo sleeve! Suddenly, I felt like a rebel with a cause: the cause of having some fun!

Diane instructed me that I must slather lotion on my arm every day. She explained because of the lymphedema, the integrity of my skin was at risk. She cautioned me to be wary of cuts, scratches, and insect bites, as they could quickly cause an infection.

Diane asked me to return to the massage bed because it was time for my lymphatic massage instructions. She stressed it was important I follow the step-by-step directions daily. Diane explained the purpose was to retrain my lymph nodes since they were confused by the missing nodes. I heard a loud pop as she pressed her thumb into my tissue. I must have looked alarmed because she said, "The pop you just heard is good. It means some of the cording is releasing."

At the end of our session, I flipped through my planner, making sure each date was written down in dark blue ink as I scheduled a month's worth of appointments. A wave of calm washed over me as I stepped into the parking lot. I felt hope renewed, ready to take on the world one appointment at a time.

***

Internet Research:

Lymphatic Drainage Massage: What it Is, Benefits & How To Do It (clevelandclinic.org)

Lymphatic drainage massage, also known as manual lymphatic drainage, is a gentle form of massage used to relieve painful swelling in your arms and legs caused by lymphedema. Lymphedema often affects people recovering from breast cancer surgery.

***

Today's Quote:

"When you have exhausted all possibilities, remember this: You haven't."

—Thomas Edison

A Note to You:

If your oncologist recommends a lymphatic massage therapist, know that it's going to be a bit awkward. They'll actually be massaging your breast as part of the treatment. I felt really uncomfortable at first, but the relief from the swelling and heaviness proved worth it. Eventually you kind of get used to it. It's not weird; it's just a necessary step to eliminate all that excess fluid. And honestly, it starts to feel pretty good after a few sessions - not in a sexual way, of course, but in a 'thank God for some relief' kind of way.

Cancer Post #19: Through the Lens: May 3rd

The excitement never stops. The following day, I went to see my retinal specialist. A year ago, cataracts were discovered in my eyes, and a surgical procedure went horribly awry, leaving me temporarily blind in my left eye. Thanks to the specialist's skilled hands, he restored my vision. However, every routine check-up brings back the unease from when I couldn't see out of my left eye.

As I sat in the exam chair on this Tuesday afternoon, the doctor confirmed the diagnosis of glaucoma and macular degeneration. Before I could even process the news, he informed me he needed to do some minor laser surgery to correct some remnants of the grievous mistake of my last physician. This unexpected news made me both wary and weary. Between this, cancer, lymphedema, and cording, I prayed out loud to God, saying, "Okay, big guy, I have all I can bear. You can stop at any time."

The doctor worked his magic laser inside my eye for ten eternal minutes. With a merciful 'done,' he surrendered the instrument, and thankfully, it was painless, quick, and successful. Immediately, I could see better. This felt like a miracle.

***

Internet Research:

Is glaucoma related to cancer? – Quick-Advices

In conclusion, based on this nationwide longitudinal study investigating the association between glaucoma and cancer development, we found that glaucoma is a risk factor for overall cancer incidence. In addition, the risk of cancer was more prominent in female glaucoma patients and those younger than 65 years.

***

Today's Quote:

"For beautiful eyes, look for the good in others; for beautiful lips, speak only words of kindness; and for poise, walk with the knowledge that you are never alone."

—Audrey Hepburn

A Note to You:

When it feels like the weight of the world is on your shoulders, let it out and tell God or the Universe that you've had enough. Don't feel silly for screaming or yelling; sometimes, we just need to release all that pent-up emotion. So go ahead, stretch your arms up high to the sky, and let it all out. Keep going until you can't help but laugh or cry. Hang in there, pink sister; there are just some of those days!

Cancer Post #20: Goodbye Sweets: May 4th

Ah, YouTube! My second home. Every morning, I pledged to do my daily routine of YouTube exercises to help my lymph nodes move out the stuck fluids. Oh, and here's a bonus tip: extra weight is like Miracle Grow for lymphedema. So, goodbye, my sweets – I will miss you.

***

Internet Research:

Obesity and lymphedema: Connections and more (medicalnewstoday.com)

Obesity is a common condition that results in excessive fat accumulation in the body. Obesity is a significant risk factor for many conditions, including lymphedema.

***

Today's Quote:

"I'm here today because I refused to be unhappy. I took a chance."

—Wanda Sykes

A Note to You:

I keep hoping for the day they discover obesity and sweets are healthy. Sometimes, it feels as if all we do is deny ourselves, but I don't know how to change that. Maybe a giant sundae will be the new superfood. Who knows! We can dream, right?

Cancer Post #21: Popeye and Olive Oyl: May 9th

My specially made compression sleeves for lymphedema arrived, and I thought the tattoo sleeve looked groovy. As I attempted to put it on as instructed by my therapist, an overwhelming sense of self-consciousness washed over me. I didn't want to wear it publicly; it felt like a bright neon sign flashing, "Cancer victim, cancer victim."

However, I also wanted to get control over the lymphedema. My therapist reminded me to wear the garment all day and evening and only take it off when sleeping. The material was both smooth and pinchy simultaneously. The fat in my arm bulged, giving me the silhouette of a Popeye cartoon character gone bad. Only one person mentioned my sleeve all day, and she said, "Cool tattoo."

I had expected the compression sleeve to be hot and uncomfortable, but to my surprise, it was quite comfortable. The gentle pressure relieved the swelling and pain in my arm. A few days later, as I looked at my arm, I noticed it no longer resembled Popeye's muscular arm, but had a slimmer silhouette more like Olive Oyl's. This comparison resonated with me - while Olive Oyl may have been assertive and confident, she held onto feelings of cowardice. And that's precisely how I felt while facing breast cancer and all its challenges.

The compression garment shields and supports the body, elevating one's quality of life to its utmost potential. With the sleeve on, I could experience life in its finest form such as going to work without pain or worry. In mere days, I was able to relish time in my cherished flower garden. The sleeve enabled me to enjoy every precious moment to its fullest extent.

My jaw dropped as I learned the total cost: $358.67 for two compression sleeves? Medical expenses had no limit! Thankfully, my friend Kim informed me that some insurance companies cover such costs as part of their medical compression garment benefits. I would call my insurance company to see what they offered. While it pained me to spend this amount, I was grateful for the help of the compression sleeves.

***

Internet Research:

Compression sleeves for lymphedema: Types, tips, and more (medicalnewstoday.com)

A compression sleeve for lymphedema is a tube-shaped elasticized garment that a person wears on the arm. By putting pressure on the arm, it keeps lymph flowing through the lymphatic system.

***

Today's Quote:

"Keeping your body healthy is an expression of gratitude to the whole cosmos — the trees, the clouds, everything."

—Thích Nhất Hạnh

A Note to You:

As I confided in my dear friend Mary about the financial burden of my sleeve, she surprised me with a kind gesture. She and her husband sent a card and enclosed a check to cover the cost of one of my compression sleeves. Her generosity moved me deeply, especially since I had just discovered that my insurance would not cover the expense. A few months later, I met a receptionist who wore a tattered sleeve on her arm from lymphedema caused by breast cancer surgery. Her story struck a chord within me, and I couldn't stop thinking about her struggles. The next day, I slipped a check into a card and handed it to her, hoping she would be at the desk to receive it. Walking away, I felt fulfilled knowing I could make a difference in someone else's life. If you have the means, I encourage you to join Mary's Movement and pay it forward to those who may need a helping hand in their own battle with lymphedema after breast cancer surgery. Let us spread Mary's initial kindness like ripples in water, bringing hope to others who have fallen victim to this side effect. May Mary's Movement continue to march forward with love and compassion for all those affected by lymphedema.

NOTES AND THOUGHTS

CHAPTER EIGHT

LESSONS

Cancer Post #22: Revelations from the School of Life: May 13th

Amidst the constant barrage of negativity in the media, my battle with cancer revealed a hidden truth to me - that there are still countless kind souls and empathetic hearts in this world. Through sickness and struggle, I learned an invaluable lesson: humanity is full of diverse and compassionate individuals, and this realization is something I yearn for everyone to encounter. Though I wouldn't wish my illness on anyone, it opened my eyes to the overwhelming goodness within people.

There are a variety of individuals in my life-- family, friends, strangers--and each person brings his or her unique personality and background. They have all contributed to my journey in a meaningful way. I'm grateful for the love, support, gifts, prayers, positive energy, and healing I've received from this diverse group of people. They reinforced my belief that people are inherently good and amazing.

If someone you know has cancer, but you are not sure what to do, for him or her my cancer research today includes nineteen suggestions from MD Anderson.

***

Internet Research:

https://www.mdanderson.org/cancerwise/19-ways-to-help-someone-with-cancer

Want to help a friend or loved one dealing with cancer? It can be hard to know exactly what you can or should do.

***

Today's Quote:

"I don't think of all the misery but of the beauty that still remains."

—Anne Frank

A Note to You:

I know it's difficult to accept help when you've always been the one taking care of everyone else. But people want to be there for you. Here are some suggestions you can give your friends:

• Come Visit, but call first.

• Listen.

• Pray.

• Help, if you see the laundry needs folding, start folding.

• Tell a joke.

• Send messages, via text, Facebook, email, or send cards.

• Mop and vacuum their house.

• Take them a meal.

• Help with their children, pets, or plants.

• Drive them to an appointment or take them for a ride.

• Hugs.

• Be positive around them.

- Help fundraise for them if needed.

- Bring them a little gift.

- Give their caregivers a break.

- Be there.

A Note to You:

Give your friends this list or make your own, and let them take some of the burden off your shoulders. You don't have to do it all on your own. And once you feel better, pay it forward and help someone else in need. That's what sisterhood is all about.

Cancer Post #23: Get Out of Town: May 20th

If you're struggling, feel stressed, or depressed, get out of town! I zipped up my suitcase, grabbed some snacks, and jumped in the car. As my fiancé drove us down the Interstate, I felt a weight lift off my shoulders. For the first time in months, I was free from the looming doctor's appointments and scary scans. The sun shone brightly through wispy clouds as we took to the open road. Cancer worries melted away as we made memories that would last a lifetime.

Friday started off with a happy dance. My great-grandson made his appearance in the world. However, a cloud shadowed this joy because he arrived earlier than anticipated and faced difficulties. Nevertheless, he possessed the resilient Stutchman family genetics. Although concerned, I knew he would conquer these obstacles, just like other determined members of our family members before him.

Neil and I made our way to Allen, Texas, for yet another cause for celebration. His grandson, Brayden, would graduate from High School with his proud class of 1,709 students who had bravely battled the pandemic and social unrest together.

When we arrived at Brayden's pre-graduation party, my heart swelled with joy. My bonus grandson stood before me, beaming a smile so bright it could have lit the entire town. For once, cancer did not overwhelm every thought—this day was all about Brayden's momentous achievement.

As the sun set on graduation day, my heart swelled with admiration and awe for each student's determined face. Despite facing difficult circumstances, they refused to be beaten and showed incredible resilience. My pride grew as I watched them confidently stride across the stage towards a promising future.

The next day, I indulged in retail therapy at the bustling Allen Outlet Mall. Excitement bubbled within me as I made a beeline for the Cabi store. Trying on outfit after outfit, I felt like nothing could stop me and that cancer was just a temporary bump in the road. As I twirled and posed in front of the mirror, visions of all the adventures these new clothes would accompany me on filled my mind. This shopping trip reinvigorated my strength and determination to conquer any challenge that came my way.

Neil and I walked into the bar at the Marriott Allen Convention Center, and Kelley, our favorite bartender from Texas, greeted us warmly. She shared her story of battling cancer for seventeen years and overcoming it with her unbreakable spirit. Her positive energy radiated throughout the room, and we all enjoyed chatting. Kelley surprised us with a round of Grand Marnier and Hershey's chocolates, which we happily savored. While we were talking, the man next to me told me of a colossal baseball card trading show going on all weekend in the hotel and convention center. We discussed his love of baseball cards and how they have made a comeback over the years. I shared with him about my son's collection of 1980s baseball cards. This unexpected conversation brought us all joy, and the reprieve from discussing cancer energized me.

We attended my granddaughter Abby's play on Saturday evening. She stole the show with her performance as Goldilocks, and it warmed my heart to see her siblings, Adam and Ara, radiating with pride from the crowd. Afterward, we treated my son to a special birthday dinner, where the service was impeccable. Platter after platter of food arrived at our table. I indulged without reservation until my stomach reminded my brain that it could not stretch farther.

Sunday morning, the final day of our escape from reality, we shared breakfast with Neil's daughter and two grandsons, Brayden and Zak. Brayden animatedly spoke about his future ambitions, the conversation peppered with laughter and joy, amplified by the delicious spread before us. The boys devoured their food with ravenous hunger, reminding me how voracious teenagers can be.

***

Internet Research:

https://health.clevelandclinic.org/should-i-go-on-vacation-when-im-being-treated-for-cancer

You're in the middle of treatment for cancer – one of the most serious, scary and intense experiences ever. Does the idea of going on a vacation trip seem somewhat frivolous? If you're a cancer patient, taking a vacation might be exactly what you need. So much of your daily life and mental energy can revolve around treatment and visits to the doctor. A vacation can provide a respite from all that.

***

Today's Quote:

"More than 10 million Americans are living with cancer, and they demonstrate the ever-increasing possibility of living beyond cancer."

—Sheryl Crow

A Note to You:

I suggest you take a break from whatever is causing you physical or emotional distress. It's crucial that you fully immerse yourself in each moment of your getaway and allow yourself time to rest and recharge. Your well-being is a top priority, and I encourage you to focus on self-care.

When the weight of cancer starts to feel like it is crushing you, you need to take a breath and recharge your spirit. Talk to your doctors, and if they give the nod, pack your bags and escape from all this for a bit. Visit family go on a short vacation. This is your time to put yourself first and give your mind and body a well-deserved rest. You are worthy, my dear friend. Remember to care for yourself and savor each moment of your getaway.

Cancer Post #24: Pause and Contemplate: May 29th

Yesterday, my family and I gathered in my hometown to decorate the graves of our loved ones. As we lovingly placed flowers around their tombstones, the harsh reality of life's brevity hit me hard. My sister and I are both breast cancer survivors, a reminder of how fragile our time on this earth can be. Standing at our mother's grave, who lost her battle with breast cancer, I felt compelled to pay tribute to all of our family members who were taken from us too soon by this devastating disease. Later, we attended a Celebration of Life for George, a dear friend who had married into our family. His passing served as another reminder to cherish every moment we have with those we love.

I am grateful for the advances and research in cancer treatments, and my sister and I are still standing and having life adventures. However, when faced with an illness that forces you to think about the fact you could die, that same thought also makes you want to remember others in your family who battled cancer but lost. It may sound morbid, but in actuality, it is quite beautiful and may cause a smile or two or a chuckle as you remember their stories.

Our mother, Anna Marjorie Malicote, died of breast cancer in 1997. She was a fashion diva and always had friends and family over on weekends for parties or trips to the lake. Our red brick home was spotless due to her hard work. She taught me I could do anything if I worked for it and believed in myself.

At the age of 38, Phyliss Ann Stutchman Dierksen passed away from breast cancer. Those who were fortunate enough to know her recall her kind heart, Shirley Temple-esque curls, and authentic affection for others. She made sure every moment brimmed with love and happiness.

Lois Marie Stutchman died from colon cancer on September 5th, 1997, at 76. Anyone who ever sat at her kitchen table ate and ate and ate. She always prepared a feast of delicious home-cooked meals and served them with plenty of sweet tea. She sacrificed much for her family and gave selflessly to them.

May 1st, 1985, marked the day that lung cancer took Jack Stutchman's life. He moved to California at 17 and completed his education there, building a successful career. But beyond his professional achievements, he found true happiness in his wife, Elona, and their three children: Michael, Brian, and Elaine.

Cancer claimed Brian Winkler's life on April 23rd, 2006, when he was just 28 years old. Although his wife April and daughter Eva meant everything to him, he also had a passion for Oklahoma University football. Not only did

Brian pass all four sections of the CPA exam on his first try, but he also never failed to have a contagious smile and share a few jokes with those around him. Losing this incredible man to cancer at such a young age was an indescribable tragedy.

After decorating the graves, we sped from Enid to Oklahoma City for George's Celebration of Life. George lost his battle with brain cancer at sixty-eight. He was a renowned animal lover, even keeping a pet buffalo that loved cuddling and kissing. As loved ones shared memories of George, laughter filled the room, just as he would have wanted it. His wife Cindy assured us he was there in spirit, joining the merriment. And while he may no longer be with us, his legacy lives on through his children, Natalie and Tommy, who will continue to share tales of George for generations to come.

Cancer has plagued my family for generations. My ancestors bravely battled it, leaving a legacy of fortitude and determination. Little did they know that their struggles would pave the way for ongoing research and the discovery of life-saving treatments for my sister, myself, and countless others. I am grateful for their unwavering courage and grace amid this cruel disease.

***

Internet Research:

Is Breast Cancer Hereditary? Genetic Risk in Families (clevelandclinic.org)

Genes that can raise your risk for breast cancer can be passed through the generations on either side of your family tree.

***

Today's Quote:

"Take time to be thankful for today, for tomorrow is never a guarantee."

—Shelley Stutchman, Author of *PEEK-A-BOOB* and Breast Cancer Survivor

A Note to You:

I struggled to write this post, but happiness filled my heart as I reminisced about the people I mentioned. It made me realize how crucial it is to document and share our experiences with our loved ones. Imagine how priceless it would be to read a letter from a deceased family member telling their life story. So, pick up that pen or open your laptop and start writing. This will be one of the greatest legacies you can leave for future generations and researchers. And if you need more time to be ready to write everything out, treat yourself to a beautiful notebook and jot down notes of the stories you want to live on years after you've passed to the other side.

Cancer Post #25: Sisterly Chronicles: May 30th

My sister and breast cancer survivor, Willow LaMunyon, wrote this post.

***

I avoided writing about breast cancer until Shelley finished the easy part. Tests, surgeries, treatments that make a person sick, knowing people are poisoning you to cure you, physical discomfort, emotional trauma, and frightening medical equipment are the easy parts. You must wonder if I have completely lost it to call that the easy part. I have not.

Like Shelley, I have been there and know the feelings she has been and will be experiencing. There is waking up in the night feeling the terror that it will be back and tearing apart your body even more. There is worrying that you may be enjoying the most positive attention you have ever received in your life and that attention might be addictive, and you will want to be sick to keep it going.

A strange twinge might be a symptom of cancer returning, or it could be a sign of becoming a hypochondriac. Not knowing if an emergency room visit is in order or ignoring it quickly becomes obsessive.

Your body doesn't feel the same as it did before—it doesn't even feel like your own body. You don't know how your body will respond, and you can't determine what you can or can't do.

You're a different person. Physically and especially emotionally, you are no longer the person you were.

Sometimes, there is the elation of having survived, and the world becomes more beautiful and every day more precious. There are, personal promises to become a better, stronger person and thinking I am new, now fresh born into a wiser me. Maybe there was a reason to have experienced cancer. Perhaps it was a good thing, an eye-opener.

Life can be such a paradox. The elation has another side, and it is called anger. You have become a different person and started to explore the new you. The new you becomes yet again a different you, and you can't stop thinking and talking about your breast cancer. Your own mind feels like a movie plot that doesn't make sense. Thank goodness for antidepressants and a medical staff that knows how to help.

***

Internet Research:

The Risk of Suicide in Cancer Patients (verywellhealth.com)

According to a 2019 study, suicide is most common in the first 3 months after someone is diagnosed with cancer. With an overall risk twice that of the general population, this risk can be as much as 13 times the average suicide risk in those newly diagnosed with cancer.

***

Today's Quote:

"When we long for life without difficulties, remind us that oaks grow strong in contrary winds, and diamonds are made under pressure."

—Peter Marshall

A Note to You:

When my sister pointed out that you might feel guilty for enjoying the attention of having cancer, it really hit home for me. I'll admit, I've had moments where I relished in the extra attention, even played the cancer card, and then questioned myself, "What kind of weirdo am I?"

But here's the thing - it's okay to give yourself a break and accept the perks that come with being a cancer patient. We go through so much. We deserve some special treatment. As you become stronger and healthier, that feeling of needing extra attention will fade, so don't worry about it too much. Embrace the love and care that comes your way. You deserve it all.

Knowledge allows for preparation to overcome the emotional trauma related to breast cancer. Here is the list written by my sister, Willow LaMunyon.

***

• Get professional help through antidepressants, counseling, or both. Your doctor will probably talk to you about it even before you ask. I have survived breast cancer for over 30 years, but I still take antidepressants. My doctor changes them now and then to prevent addiction and ensure they continue working.

• In-person breast cancer support groups help keep survivors informed and allow them to relax with others experiencing the same things. A good group will provide all kinds of fun and information. Often, lifetime friendships come from those groups.

• Continued support of family and friends for the long haul is important beyond all else. Life will again start making sense again. So slowly, it is easy to go unnoticed as all the pieces of life begin to fit together again, and you discover that the you that you were born with is still there but stronger, wiser, braver, and happy.

NOTES AND THOUGHTS

Chapter Nine
RADIATION

Cancer Post #26: Trepidation and Joy: May 31st

With only eighteen days until our wedding, I felt joy. However, my specialized radiation operation taking place in three days put a wet blanket on my enthusiasm. Talk about poor timing. Despite my pleas to reschedule earlier or postpone until after the wedding, the radiologist refused. Cutting it close doesn't even begin to describe it. Everything had been planned and paid for months in advance - invitations sent, venues booked, food ordered, photographer arranged, and the DJ scheduled. No rescheduling at this point. The nuclear physicians' schedule coincided with this narrow time frame, leaving me stuck.

Optimism, however, helped offset the scheduling problem. Even though the surgeon believed they got all the cancer when they removed the tumor, the radiation would be a safety net. But I grappled with the fear of a potential recurrence. I tried to trust in God and banish worry, yet I still fretted. The urge to unwind with a couple of glasses of wine beckoned until I remembered the research I found linking wine and cancer. I resisted indulging.

***

Internet Research:

Drinking Alcohol (breastcancer.org)

Research consistently shows that drinking alcoholic beverages — beer, wine, and liquor — increases a woman's risk of hormone-receptor-positive breast cancer. Alcohol can increase levels of estrogen and other hormones associated with hormone-receptor-positive breast cancer. Alcohol also may increase breast cancer risk by damaging DNA in cells.

Compared to women who don't drink at all, women who have three alcoholic drinks per week have a 15% higher risk of breast cancer. Experts estimate that the risk of breast cancer goes up another 10% for each additional drink women regularly have each day.

***

Today's Quote:

"Wine a little and you'll feel better."

—Anonymous

A Note to You:

This research about wine and its connection to breast cancer left me confused. I loved sipping on a nice glass of wine in the evenings, but I questioned whether it was worth the potential health risks. I decided to cut back and alternate between drinking days and abstinence days. It was tough because I didn't want to give up something I enjoyed, but I also didn't want to jeopardize my health. What do you think? Have you talked to your doctor about this if you're also a wine lover? I'd hate for either of us to miss our beloved vino, but we must prioritize our well-being.

Cancer Post #27: Eureka Moments: May 31st

With my top half exposed, I climbed onto the exam table with my left arm behind my neck as I waited for the Ultrasound to commence. The chill in the room made me shiver and I asked for a blanket. Miraculously, a lovely, warm one soon arrived afterward, providing me with much comfort. As the testing began, so did my racing thoughts. The technician speaking in the sweetest Southern drawl distracted me from my anxiousness, and I started chatting with her. Suddenly, in mid-sentence, I heard another voice inside my head telling me, "Stop talking, Shelley! Don't distract her from her work."

She finished the procedure and, with her Southern twang, said, "I will be right back with the doctor to read the results." She added, "Oh, and don't put back on your clothes just yet." By now, I had gotten used to being topless.

I breathed a sigh of relief and felt my nerves calm down, but my relief was short-lived as the radiologist and technician entered with serious expressions. I must have looked scared because the doctor reassured me, "Don't worry, it's just a seroma. It's not cancerous, just some fluid."

A seroma? Of course, rather than ask the doctor for more clarification, I waited until I could pull out my phone and ask Dr. Google. I found out a seroma is a build-up of clear bodily fluids in a place on your body where tissue has been removed by surgery. I learned most seromas are reabsorbed back into your body in about a month, but in some cases, it can take up to a year.

***

Internet Research:

Seroma formation after surgery for breast cancer | World Journal of Surgical Oncology Full Text (biomedcentral.com)

Seroma formation is the most frequent postoperative complication after breast cancer surgery. It occurs in most patients after mastectomy and is now increasingly being considered a side effect of surgery rather than a complication.

***

Today's Quote:

"Once you choose hope, anything's possible."

—Christopher Reeve

A Note to You:

My heart dropped as I felt my body once again betraying me. "Not another side effect," I muttered through clenched teeth.

It felt so unfair. Life had already dealt me the cancer card; why did it have to keep piling on more health issues? I knew this seroma wasn't serious, but it was just one more thing to deal with, and I felt like I was at my breaking point.

But then I realized these were just negative thoughts, "stinkin' thinkin'." It wasn't cancer, and for that, I should be grateful. Maybe all these side effects were happening so I could use them as teachable moments. This positive thinking helped me feel better than my initial reaction of "Oh no, here we go again."

I know it can feel overwhelming when buried under a mountain of side effects. But hang in there, friend. Those side effects will eventually become less and less and someday feel like a distant memory. When that time comes, reach out your hand to others who are struggling. We're in this together.

Cancer Post #28: Reflections on the Eve of Surgery: May 31st

On Wednesday morning, I would undergo a Multicatheter HDR Interstitial Brachytherapy procedure. Brachyther-apy allowed for the temporary placement of small radioactive seeds within the breast targeted in the area at the highest risk of residual cancer. I'm impressed by how fluently I can spout out medical terms now.

The catheter placement would take place at the hospital and would take approximately ninety minutes. At the completion of the catheter placement, the radiologist would apply plastic buttons to the ends of the tubes to secure them in place. To minimize the risk of infection, antibiotic ointment would be applied to my wounds.

The following week, I started my radiation treatment plan. The plan involved five days of twice-daily treatments in a room with only a table and essential tools. During each session, my radiologist and two physicists meticulously mapped the distribution of radioactive seeds into the catheters inserted into my left breast connected to a machine. Another physicist would be on standby, monitoring the procedure. After each treatment, I would be free of any nuclear material and pose no threat to the people around me.

After each session, a nurse would change my dressings and apply lidocaine to numb the area surrounding the catheter placement. I was also prescribed Keflex to take three times daily to prevent infection. Lastly, Oxycodone had been prescribed for pain relief.

I felt fortunate to have been deemed eligible for this therapy. I'm grateful I didn't have to undergo the five weeks of radiotherapy, which would have happened if I had not qualified for Brachytherapy. Brachytherapy significantly reduces the risk of side effects on the patient's heart, lungs, and skin from radiation.

***

Internet Research:

https://my.clevelandclinic.org/health/treatments/16500-brachytherapy

Brachytherapy is a highly effective treatment for certain types of cancer. It's most effective on cancers that haven't spread, or metastasized. Most side effects improve as the radiation leaves your body.

***

Today's Quote:

"Every negative belief weakens the partnership between mind and body."

—Deepak Chopra

A Note to You:

There are a ton of options available for radiation treatments. Ask your radiologist to explain all the types you qualify for. Don't let the doctors pressure you to decide on the spot. Take your time and do some research before making a choice. I know it can feel overwhelming, but being well-informed is key to taking control of your treatment plan. Plus, consider all the knowledge you'll gain to pass on to others in similar situations.

Cancer Post #29: Unexpected Workplace Prescription: June 1st

The day of my surgery I received a text from my boss, Cathy. She said she was praying for me, which was appreciated, but that's not all! As an RN, she reminded me to use a stool softener - shocker! In my sixty-seven years, I never had a boss who cared so much she'd remind me to take a laxative - how funny! My boss started my day off with a chuckle. Laughter is the best medicine to settle nerves.

***

Today's research lesson:

Constipation From Opioid Painkillers (webmd.com)

Medications called opioids can knock out some of the toughest pain. But they can also make you constipated. The problem doesn't always start right away. It can happen any time you're taking the drug. Your best bet is to try to keep the problem from happening. When your doctor gives you a prescription for an opioid, ask about ways you can avoid constipation. If it does happen, ask your doctor about treatment. Call them right away if you feel severe pain.

Unlike other side effects from these drugs, like feeling sleepy or nauseated, constipation doesn't go away after a few days on the medication. Scientists think this is because your gut doesn't get used to opioids the way the rest of your body does. The longer you take the drug, the bigger the chance it will block you up.

***

Today's Quote:

"This poo shall pass."

—Anonymous

A Note to You:

Listen, sweetie, trust me when I say constipation is no joke. I learned the hard way during my strict Keto diet days. So, here's the deal: stay hydrated like a freakin' camel, load up on those fruits and veggies like they're going out of style, get your daily dose of fiber (think bran flakes, not cardboard), and keep some laxatives handy just in case those surgeries or meds try to slow down your bowel party. You'll thank me later. Trust me, I've been there.

Cancer Post #30: Surgery was Fun: June 1st

Yes, you read my headline correctly. I enjoyed myself during my surgery. Throughout the procedure, I stayed awake and twisted into all sorts of crazy positions as they inserted the catheter tubes in my left breast. The doctor numbed the area and gave me a cocktail of Valium and Oxycodone. With that mixture of pills, the world bloomed with color and euphoria for me.

From the moment the pills took effect, I felt a deep connection with my doctor, physicists, nurses, and techs. We were like old buddies who had grown up together. I yammered endlessly throughout the entire ninety-minute surgery. Each word that came flying out of my mouth seemed more brilliant and funnier than the last. At one point, I even asked the radiologist how much dough she made each year. Her reply? "Let's just say I do alright."

The doctor kept asking me if I was okay. In response, I kept giggling and trying to figure out how they were weaving those catheter tubes through my breast. The procedure fascinated me. The whir of so many people looking at my breast seemed hilarious. The smell of disinfectant permeated the room with its tangy aroma that, under the cocktail of drugs, I thought smelled terrific. This operation was unlike any process I had ever seen before because even though I was drugged up, I was awake and watching and hearing the medical team talk. Magic.

I felt like a detached observer as I watched the surgeons and nurses bustling around me. My left breast was covered in clear catheter tubes, stretching out like delicate peacock feathers. The sight had a strange beauty to it. "Do you mind if I take a picture?" I asked the nurse.

She chuckled and nodded, amused. "I snuck my phone in," I confessed with a laugh, pointing to an inconspicuous bulge under my right buttock.

The nurse rummaged under the sheet like she was searching for buried treasure and finally pulled out my phone from its designated spot. The physicist had performed some magical transformation on my catheter tubes, turning them into patriotic red, white, and blue decorations sticking out of my chest.

As I begged for more photos, everyone in the room howled with laughter—at least, that's what I imagined in my altered state, and I became the funniest person in the world—in my mind. I knew I'd get a call from Comedy Central any day now.

The surgery was called Ultrasound Guided Interstitial Radioelement. The purpose was to prepare my breast for brachytherapy. The radiologist strategically slid long needles from one side of my breast to the other. After completing the insertion, she slipped the flexible catheters over the needles, and I felt pressure as she pushed open my skin to make them fit. There were eighteen catheter tubes in all. Each tube had an insertion point and an exit point. In total, thirty-six incisions were made in my left breast. Once the tubes were in, buttons were attached to my breast to hold everything in place. I couldn't feel it when the doctor pulled out the needles from the tubes. I guess you could call her a smooth operator. Next, the team ensured the catheter tubes were open to allow the radioactive seeds insertion. The physicist then capped the lines and numbered them. Different strengths of radiation would go into each tube. The surgery ended when the nurse applied a sterile dressing to my left breast.

The valium and oxycontin cocktail continued working its magic. Sitting in recovery with me, Neil asked, "How was the surgery, and how do you feel?"

I replied with a chuckle, "It was absolutely amazing! If I had known how great it would be, I never would have been so nervous!" Then I added, "The world is so beautiful, and you are beautiful, and I'm beautiful."

When we arrived home, I wanted to eat. I sipped on the tomato soup Neil prepared as if it were ambrosia from the gods. Everything around me still glimmered and sparkled - even mundane objects like a toothbrush or cup filled me with sheer joy. I've never tried ecstasy, but I imagine it is what people experience when they take that drug.

I drifted off into a peaceful sleep until a sharp jolt of agony shot up my spine. Taking no time to recover from the shock, I forced myself to stand and drag myself from the bed to the couch—hoping that changing positions would provide relief. In the eerie darkness of four in the morning, I reached for my phone and scrolled through messages. I paused when I noticed a post from my friend Claudette. I texted back to her I was in pain, not expecting her to be awake. But Claudette quickly replied with a powerful prayer that seemed to echo through me. Miraculously, the pain evaporated as soon as I finished reading her message. A deep sense of awe washed over me. In equal measure, I thanked her and God and settled back into a blissful slumber.

As the morning sun rose, I arrived at the Cancer Center for my wound dressing appointment. The radiology team greeted me warmly and tended to my needs, making me feel valued and cared for.

***

Today's Cancer Research:

Brachytherapy for Cancer - NCI

Brachytherapy is a type of internal radiation therapy in which seeds, ribbons, or capsules that contain a radiation source are placed in your body, in or near the tumor. Brachytherapy is a local treatment and treats only a specific part of your body. It is often used to treat cancers of the head and neck, breast, cervix, prostate, and eye.

***

Today's Quote:

"Values are related to our emotions, just as we practice physical hygiene to preserve our physical health, we need to observe emotional hygiene to preserve a healthy mind and attitudes."

—Dalai Lama

A Note to You:

Girl, don't you think it's crazy how some meds can make us totally loopy? I swear, I had the wildest experience with them. I even started bragging to my medical team, "Aren't you all lucky to have such a smart patient like me? I may even be smarter than some of you!"

And let me tell you, feeling that smart made me feel like a total boss. Especially since I've done so much research about cancer and treatments - knowledge is power! So next time you have surgery, just remember, my pink sister, the more you know about your illness, the more powerful you are.

Cancer Post #31: Gas: June 2nd

Yes, this is a post about gas. Not the type they call flatus, but the overpriced kind. We were driving to the hospital to get my dressing changed. We filled up our tank despite the cost, even though we complained about the high price. We have a reliable car. It made me ponder how cancer patients who don't have the money for the millions of trips they have to make for treatments or reliable transportation make it work.

I asked my attending medical professional what would happen to those unable to finance the costs of traveling to and from treatment. The nurse answered that the facility established a foundation to provide individuals with free gas cards for those who qualify. For people living in more rural areas, they also offered hotel accommodations. "What about patients without their own vehicle?" I asked.

Her eyes welled with tears as she recounted the answer to my question. She explained how the staff go above and beyond to ensure their patients have access to life-saving treatments, even donating their own money, if necessary, to pay for an Uber ride if a patient is in need. Her quiet reverence as she spoke of her colleagues' generosity moved everyone in the room.

The nurse changed my dressing. Her hands were gentle but efficient. "How are you feeling?" she asked.
I squirmed a little, trying to adjust the heavy contraption woven into my breast. It felt like having someone wrap their fingers too tightly around your arm—you can feel it, and it's uncomfortable but not painful. I glanced down, embarrassed by how lopsided I looked. My left breast was more than twice the size of my right one.

I napped at least twice daily. I asked my nurse why this was happening when I hadn't even started radiation. Her response boiled down to the catheter surgery, pain meds, and the emotional strain of having cancer draining me of any energy. Ugh, I hated being so tired all the time! There was so much to do, but no get-up-and-go to get it done! This was SO frustrating!

***

Internet Research:

Komen Financial Assistance Program - Susan G. Komen®

Financial hardships shouldn't keep those with breast cancer from getting the care they need. While medical treatment and care are typically the primary costs associated with a breast cancer diagnosis, there are other expenses of daily living that can prevent patients from getting the care they need, when they need it. The Komen Financial Assistance Program is here to help. Go to their website and apply for financial assistance programs, including those for prescription drugs and other medical costs, transportation, lodging, and child and elder care.

***

Today's Quote:

"Don't be afraid to ask for help; seeking financial advice is a sign of strength, not weakness."

—Anonymous

A Note to You:

My dear friend, dealing with illness often brings unexpected financial burdens. It can be daunting to reach out for help from agencies, but they are there for a reason and will handle things discreetly. If you need assistance, don't hesitate to take it. And when you're back on your feet, pay it forward. You have enough on your plate without worrying about money. Support always.

Cancer Post #32: Navigating Challenges with Valium: June 3rd

In the depths of this post, I will strip away all layers and expose my soul to you. My promise to be unflinchingly honest and vulnerable about my journey through breast cancer is one I hold dear. Anyone undergoing the same struggles, deserves nothing less than my wholehearted transparency.

An unfathomable despair consumed me last night. My left breast throbbed relentlessly, the tiny plastic tubes inside me torturing my skin with incessant itching. I longed to rip them out and end this cancer journey once and for all. With every fiber of my being, I begged the deity above for mercy - heal me or take me home. The limbo was unbearable, and I believed I couldn't endure it any longer.

I battled with conflicting versions of myself, one fading while the other struggled to emerge. This phase magnified into a constant source of unease, akin to a bad haircut that required time to grow out. Despite my longing for a cure bringing me back to full health, I couldn't ignore the fact pain and discomfort were inevitable parts of the journey.

Exhaustion seeped into every fiber of my being, and the weight of work left unfinished on my desk bore down on me. I believed this was Karma's way of punishing me for all the times I had carelessly hurt others. The temptation to wallow in self-pity crept over me. But then, my analytical side snapped into action, reminding me many others faced far greater challenges than I faced. I needed to shake off my self-centered state and move forward.

While I was still working, a few days prior to starting radiation treatment, I received a package filled with various bottles of pills. As I opened it, my jaw dropped in surprise at the sight of a bottle of Valium hidden among the other medications. I grumbled about not needing any antidepressants. My boss, Cathy, walked over to me and gently spoke, her forehead creased with concern. "Perhaps they included the Valium because they know what lies ahead for you. It's there just in case you need it."

My composure threatened to shatter as I fought to keep a smile plastered on my lips. The doctor's audacity, prescribing Valium without my consent, sent rage coursing through me. But I bit back my words and hid my boiling anger.

Childhood memories of my mother's dependence on valium stormed through my mind. Doctors prescribed it to calm my mother's nerves, but it became her worst enemy. She couldn't function without that tiny yellow pill, trapped in an addiction she couldn't escape. As a young child, I watched helplessly as she dozed off for hours on the couch, unable to do anything but sleep. The sight of her struggling only filled me with fear and helplessness. One day, around ten years of age, I climbed onto the couch next to her napping form, hugging her, and vowing never to fall victim to a pill that would make me sleep through life. But despite her efforts to get professional help, my mother's addiction only worsened until no choice remained but to be admitted to a mental health facility. Even then, long-term recovery was an uphill battle.

That night, when trying to fall asleep, I recalled my boss's words about my medical team knowing what they were doing. Anxiety flooded my body, and I was desperate for relief. I grabbed the pill bottle from my bedside table and shook out a small yellow tablet. Picking up a glass of water, I swallowed it before collapsing onto my pillow. Before long, the darkness of sleep carried me away.

I dedicated some time to watching YouTube videos on breast cancer and depression. It was eye-opening to discover that many women experience moments of profound emotional turmoil as they grapple with the harsh reality of having a potentially life-threatening disease.

My boss, Cathy, consistently offered valuable advice. I held her words in high regard when she assured me that my care team was highly competent. I decided to reserve the use of Valium for situations where I believed it was absolutely essential for pain relief or calming out-of-control anxiety. I've realized that this medication might offer some much-needed assistance during the upcoming week, with the twice-a-day radiation treatments or when the urge to pull the catheter tubes from my breast became overpowering. No refill option came with the Valium. I wouldn't become addicted.

I greeted the morning after my first good night's sleep in weeks. Neil and I grabbed our steaming mugs of coffee and settled onto the porch. I looked up in awe at the glorious colors peeking over the horizon and smiled with gratitude for another sunrise. Our flower garden blazed with vibrant hues reminding me of how beautiful life can be.

***

Internet Research:

Valium to Manage Anxiety Disorders and Symptoms (verywellmind.com)

Valium is a drug used for managing anxiety disorders and short-term treatment of anxiety symptoms. The drug, which is also sold under the generic name diazepam, works by actually slowing down activity in your brain.

Valium can help people who need relief from anxiety, but it can also have side effects and risks you should understand before you begin taking this medication.

***

Today's Quote:

"In three words I can sum up everything I've learned about life: It goes on."

—Robert Frost

A Note to You:

I want to have a serious conversation with you about your prescribed medications. As someone who has witnessed the destructive impact of addiction firsthand, I beg you to use caution and closely monitor any medication for anxiety and pain management. While they may provide temporary relief during our darkest moments, relying on them too heavily can lead to dependency. Promise yourself before taking one to talk to your doctor immediately if you sense yourself slipping into that trap. Your well-being means everything to your health and to your family and friends. Let's stay vigilant and make sure these meds don't numb us from fully experiencing life. You and I are in this together, my pink sister.

Cancer Post #33: Bathe, Saran Wrap, and The Total Woman: June 4th

Everyone at the cancer center vehemently warned me, "Under no circumstances should you get your left breast and the tubes wet!"

I was afraid to bathe. After not showering or bathing for a few days, I could smell myself—not a pleasing aroma, either. I knew I must get creative and get this stink washed off me without causing infection to the open areas in my skin.

I literally scratched my head in bewilderment, pondering how to safely "scrub away" my odor. It's funny how our minds can wander to unexpected places. I thought about Mirabel Morgan's literary gem of 1975, The Total Woman, which gave tips to wives of the era on how to make their marriages come alive.

It was 1975, and I was on a mission to be the perfect wife. So, I eagerly bought the book, devoured its pages, highlighted key tips, and put them into action. One particularly interesting tip caught my attention: greet your husband at the door wearing nothing but Saran Wrap and hand him a martini (or his drink of choice). Needless to say, it made for some interesting evenings in our household.

Eureka! Saran Wrap was my golden ticket to a luxurious soak in the tub. I wrapped my chest with layers of plastic wrap and dipped into the warm, shallow water. As I basked in the soothing sensation, I couldn't help but think perhaps a martini would complete this spa experience.

Thanks to the 1975 book by Mirabel Morgan and Saran Wrap, I no longer offended with bad odor.

***

Internet Research:

https://www.yahoo.com/lifestyle/easy-way-waterproof-phone

When you are in the middle of cancer treatments, you don't want to be without your phone. Appointment times can change, or your team needs to tell you something.

What you need: Saran Wrap.

What you do: Wrap the plastic wrap around your iPhone. One layer is enough--just be sure the charger port is covered, too.

And here's the genius part: The plastic wrap is thick enough to protect against water droplets, but thin enough that the touchscreen will still work.

***

Today's Quote:

"When in doubt take a bath."

—Mae West

A Note to You:

Lume deodorant, developed by an OB/GYN, is also an option for body order coming from our lady parts. Isn't it hilarious how our brains can randomly recall obscure information from the past and miraculously apply it to present situations? That self-help book on becoming the perfect wife definitely didn't do much for my marriage, but it gave me a solution to my bath problem. But hey, when life throws a curveball, remember to think outside the box and embrace your inner genius! Trust me, it works like a charm... most of the time.

Cancer Post #34: A Plush Haven: June 4th

It's truly remarkable how the simplest gestures can provide immense relief. A group of women from a local church created small pillows and generously donated them to my cancer center. These pillows appeared unassuming, but they fit perfectly under my arm and the best part? They were free.

I decided to take one of these pillows, which proved to be a source of incredible comfort. With eighteen catheter tubes sticking out of my breast, this little pillow became my lifeline. I tucked it snugly under my arm. It prevented chafing when I inadvertently swung my arm, and it rubbed against the emerging tubes.

This unassuming pillow became a symbol of hope, a thread of positivity I clung to throughout the radiation treatments. I thanked God for the generosity of the church ladies.

***

Internet Research:

Mastectomy Pillows For Breast Cancer Treatment (verywellhealth.com)

Mastectomy pillows protect your incisions by keeping pressure off your chest. It can also be a comfort aid while recovering from breast cancer treatment. Sometimes referred to as "comfort pillows," these specialized pillows are useful when you're in the hospital, at home, riding in the car, and in bed at night.

***

Today's Quote:

"Self-care is not selfish. You cannot serve from an empty vessel."

—Eleanor Brownn, author

A Note to You:

Take note of these selfless actions from the church ladies, my dear. It's a powerful reminder that we can be angels of mercy in our daily lives through simple acts of kindness. Let us make it our mission to spread love and compassion wherever we go.

Cancer Post #35: Fashion Armor for Modern Warriors: June 6th

I endured being trapped in a bra for twelve days. The bra held my dressings and catheters in place. Even after the treatments ended, boob imprisonment by the bra continued for two more days to ensure the coverings stayed put. My chest had thirty-six holes to heal, a number that varies from woman to woman, depending on breast size. While we often strive to be above average in life, I was grateful for my average chest in this situation.

People constantly bombard me with one question: "How did I manage to find anything to wear with those boob tubes sticking out from my chest?"

The radiation team helped me prepare for the brachytherapy by suggesting what to wear.

The Bra:

When getting a sports bra for a radiology procedure, choose one with hooks or zips in the front. The radiology team recommended buying a bra larger than your normal size. I usually wore a medium sports bra from Walmart, but I bought a large one for this procedure. I should have gone for an extra-large. Your breast will likely swell, and you will have tubes sticking out of it, along with half an inch of dressing on top of that. Learn from my mistake and choose a bra big enough to accommodate the swelling and the tubes.

The Shirt:

Wear shirts that button down the front. Once again, the radiology team suggested getting a shirt larger than your regular size. I had purchased a large, though I should have gone with an extra-large since the buttons pulled open across my left breast.

The Emotions:

While going through your treatments, it is normal to have mini and major breakdowns. The brachytherapy took its toll, causing frequent meltdowns. Seeking support, I confided in one of the physicians on my care team. His empathetic gaze met mine as he reassured me, "It's okay to have a breakdown. Cancer is a big deal both physically and emotionally."

His acknowledgment felt like a hug to my emotional well-being.

***

Internet Research:

What Is a Breast Cancer's Grade? | Grading Breast Cancer | American Cancer Society

Cancer cells are given a grade when they are removed from the breast and checked in the lab. The grade is based on how much the cancer cells look like normal cells. The grade is used to help predict your outcome (prognosis) and to help figure out what treatments might work best.

A low grade number (grade 1) usually means the cancer is slower-growing and less likely to spread. A high

grade number (grade 3) means a faster-growing cancer that's more likely to spread.

An intermediate grade number (grade 2) means the cancer is growing faster than a grade 1 cancer but slower than a grade 3 cancer.

***

Today's Quote:

"Never be ashamed of a scar. It simply means you were stronger than whatever tried to hurt you."

—Unknown

***

A Note to You

Catching my cancer early resulted in a Stage 1 Grade 2 tumor. That grade 2 kicked my butt and caused me to have more treatments. Luckily, my Facebook friend, Jane, noticed when I was feeling down and sent me some hilarious videos by Leanne Morgan. Those reels brought some much-needed laughter. So don't hesitate to ask your friends to send you funny stuff. Tell them that humor is still to be found even in the darkest times, and laughter is the best medicine. Wishing you moments of joy and laughter, my fellow pink sisters.

Cancer Post #36: Two Down: June 6th

As I underwent my first two brachytherapy radiation treatments, I felt like the star of a science fiction movie. The nurse escorted me to a dimly lit chamber. The walls loomed over me, constructed of impenetrable cement, and the door sealed tightly with an imposing weight. The room exuded an air of containment as if it held a force so potent it must be locked away from everyone—well, everyone other than the patient.

I removed my shirt and bra, and a nurse unwrapped the dressings from my swollen breast. The eighteen catheter tubes snapped upright like raised eyebrows. She connected their ends to a metal machine next to the bed. I watched in fascination. I asked, "How do the seeds get through the tubes? Do you use a liquid or air?"

The physicist took over answering my question: "Radioactive seeds at the tip of a wire are inserted into the breast tissue. One at a time, a seed is put into a catheter. The seeds stay in place for the time that has been mapped out, and then the wire extracts the seed."

She made this complicated procedure sound simple.

I gazed inquisitively at the Geiger counter on the wall. "What secrets does it guard?" I asked.

She explained that the counter was designed to measure radiation. She also mentioned that I would hear clicking sounds while the measurement was taken. The clicks are produced when radioactive particles enter the machine and cause ions and electrons to separate. The frequency of clicks I heard during the process indicated how often this occurred per minute.

The medical staff left me alone in the cold, sterile room to protect themselves from radiation. As the door shut behind the entourage of doctors, physicists, and nurses, I felt truly isolated. The only link to the outside world was a tiny camera in the corner and a speaker crackling with static from the intercom system. I felt small and insignificant in the vastness of the space. One of the nurses left me a warm blanket before she exited the room. I wrapped it around myself gratefully, feeling a comforting embrace.

I experienced a panic attack. I felt trapped in a cement coffin. When my gaze shifted to the Geiger counter, dread seized my heart. The needle had reached 467.5! Could it be true? Was I really exposed to that devastating level of radiation? What could stop it from ravaging my body? I prayed my medical team knew what they were doing.

Radiation in high doses can be extremely dangerous and can cause sickness and even death within a short period of time. After I completed the radiation treatment, I was curious about the significance of the number 467.5. I conducted research on Google and discovered that this number is related to radioactive matter. Although I am not an expert in this field and cannot verify the accuracy of my findings, here is what I discovered:

- 10,000.00 Fatal
- 6,000.00 Possible Death
- 5,000.00 Would kill half the people exposed to that level
- 1,000.00 Estimated to cause a fatal cancer many years after the exposure
- 400.00 Max radiation levels without significant side effects

Each member of my team wore a Geiger counter to check their levels of radiation exposure. When my treatment sessions were complete, a technician came in armed with a wand that emitted a loud clicking sound and scanned me from top to bottom. Once the needle settled onto zero, another staff member unclipped the wires connected to the machine, allowing me to leave.

Every day that week, I underwent radiation treatments twice a day. One benefit was a coveted parking spot. Despite enduring no physical pain, the procedure exacted a heavy toll on my mind and body. Each session lasted thirty to forty-five minutes, not including the half-hour drive each way. On Friday, June 10th, I completed all my sessions. Now, only six days of recovery stood between me and marrying the love of my life. I would walk down the aisle on Friday, June 17th.

The science of brachytherapy invoked great admiration for the brilliant minds that created this form of radiation. I am filled with gratitude, knowing I benefited from this research and treatment progress.

With the completion of my Brachytherapy, I received a much-needed break from any cancer treatments, courtesy of my compassionate doctors. It was their wedding gift to me. However, upon returning from our honeymoon, I faced a new challenge - starting a regimen of hormone blockers. The mere thought of this medication filled me with apprehension more than anything else I encountered during my battle with cancer.

***

Internet Research:

Radiation Therapy for Cancer - NCI

At high doses, radiation therapy kills cancer cells or slows their growth by damaging their DNA. Cancer cells whose DNA is damaged beyond repair stop dividing or die. When the damaged cells die, they are broken down and removed by the body.

Radiation therapy does not kill cancer cells right away. It takes days or weeks of treatment before DNA is damaged enough for cancer cells to die. Then, cancer cells keep dying for weeks or months after radiation therapy ends.

PEEK-A-BOOB

***

Today's Quote:

"Health is like money; we never have a true idea of its value until we lose it."

Josh Billings, humor writer

A Note to You:

The radiation chamber is an opportunity for transcendence. As you lay on the cold metal bed, absorb the energy of all those who have come before you radiating through your body. Connect with their spirits and send out waves of positivity to the woman who will take your place after treatment. Let our collective love and support permeate the sterile walls and create a sanctuary of healing energy. The physical may be concrete, but our minds can transform it into something beautiful and transformative.

Cancer Post #37: Sex and Radiation: June 8th

My cheeks felt hot when I asked the nurse, "This is probably an awkward question, but...you see, I'm getting married next week, and we have plans to go on our honeymoon right after...and I was wondering if there was any chance that my soon-to-be husband could contract radiation if he... er...sucked on my nipples?"

I caught a glimpse of her, almost hesitant, smile as she replied, "No one has asked me that before." We shared an awkward giggle.

The nurse clarified, "No, you're not radioactive. Your partner won't receive radiation from kissing your nipple. In Brachytherapy, all the radioactive seeds are removed after each session."

"Excellent," I said with relief. "I didn't want Neil to have a nuclear-powered smile!"

Then she added, "I would wait until July before you have him fondle you too much on your affected breast. Your left breast has endured a lot of trauma with all these treatments. You need some time to heal."

***

Internet Research:

How Can Breast Cancer Affect Sex? (webmd.com)

Keep talking to your partner. Your partner may have their own worries about sex but be reluctant to talk to you about them. They might be worried about pressuring you into sex, unsure of how you feel, and confused about where and how to touch you. They could fear your lack of desire is their fault.

When you share your concerns about sex, it could help your partner open up. Talking about it can help you and your partner feel more connected. Together, you can brainstorm ways to improve intimacy and deal with any sexual issues.

***

My Quote for today:

"You have to be willing to give up the life you planned, and instead, greet the life that is waiting for you."

—Joseph Campbell

A Note to You:

Breast cancer treatments can make it challenging to maintain a fulfilling sex life. As women, we often shy away from discussing our sexual problems. And just like talking about money, it can seem taboo to consult with your friends. Ever since my battle with breast cancer, I've noticed changes in my sexuality and intimacy with my husband. It's not easy. Reach out and hold your partner's hand to keep the spark alive. A simple squeeze can convey so much love without saying a word. Let's support each other as women and discuss our sexuality unapologetically.

NOTES AND THOUGHTS

CHAPTER TEN

BELLS

Cancer Post #38: Bells of Love and Resilience: June 10th

My heart pounded when I grasped the bell rope. It was Friday, June 10th, and after completing my last radiation therapy session, I declared myself cancer-free.

With Neil by my side, I tugged on the bell with all my might. I rang it for everyone who held significance in my life - from family and friends to coworkers and even strangers who sent prayers and positive vibes my way. My pull echoed for those still fighting cancer and served as a symbol of hope. I pulled the rope in appreciation for the gifts showered upon me during this challenging time - flowers, jewelry, wine, or a simple card. And for the messages that brought a smile to my face - cartoons, jokes, songs, anything that gave joy amidst the struggle. It was also a tribute to those who lost their battle with cancer, including my mother and loved ones: Lois, Phyllis, Jack, George, and Brian. With every clang of the bell, I poured out my gratitude for those who encouraged me to write this book.

I looked down at my chest and whispered, "Goodbye, dear Boob Tubes. We've had a wild ride these past ten days fighting off those pesky cancer cells. But now it's time for you to be immortalized in tube history. Thank you for all your hard work."

The next step involved closing the puncture sites used for administering the radiation, which typically took two to three days. Finally, I could luxuriously bathe without wrapping my chest with saran wrap.

The treatment for breast cancer is a multi-step process. The next phase would involve starting a course of medication. After about six months, reconstructive surgery would take place.

Neil designated the 10th day of each month to celebrate my triumph over cancer. His capacity for love knows no bounds. I definitely struck gold with him as my future husband.

I would miss the wonderful people on my radiation team. I loved being treated like a VIP twice a day. Being pampered and spoiled with kind words and attention from so many people opened my eyes to the importance of expressing gratitude and love daily - not just during illness. And on Friday, as I rang that bell announcing my cancer-free status, I knew I beat cancer. Sometimes, you just know.

Internet Research:

This lesson comes from the certificate presented to me by my cancer team:

While going through treatments, do it with the art of being cheerful, outstanding in high courage, tolerant, and determined in all orders given.

***

Today's Quote:

"Hope is the ability to hear the music of the future. Faith is the courage to dance to it today."

—Peter Kuzmic

A Note to You:

When you ring that bell, my sister, ring it with all your might. Let it be a celebration of triumph, like winning an Oscar or an Emmy. May the wind carry the sound of your bell far and wide, and may I somehow hear it echoing through the cosmos.

Cancer Post #39: TA: June 11th

As my friend TA, who also had cancer, said, "Ringing that bell felt like you just finished a 100k dash. A breath of fresh air filled your lungs as you knew you just completed a victory. Wow!"

***

Internet Research:

Bell ringing ritual to mark end of cancer treatment builds community, gives patients a sense of control, study finds (medicalxpress.com)

The bell-ringing ritual started at the MD Anderson Cancer Centre in Texas in 1996 and has since spread to cancer centers around the world. A patient who completes chemo or radiation treatments rings the bell, and staff and other patients cheer and take photos.

***

Today's Quote:

"Cancer changes your life, often for the better. You learn what's important, you learn to prioritize, and you learn not to waste your time. You tell people you love them."

—Joel Siegel

A Note to You:

My dear friend TA passed away before this book was published. He had requested that I include his feelings when he rang the bell. When I wrote this note, I felt TA looking down from heaven, donning his cowboy hat and holding his guitar. TA knew Toby Keith, the country singer, and I can only imagine the beautiful music they are making. Though TA didn't have breast cancer like us, all forms of cancer bring us together as brothers and sisters who have fought against it. Rest in peace, TA.

NOTES AND THOUGHTS

Chapter Eleven
WEDDING BELLS

Cancer Post #40: Love's Grand Overture: June 12th

The clock ticked relentlessly, counting down the final five days until the wedding. Through sheer determination and a fierce desire for perfection, I powered through and completed all tasks with astonishing speed. Collapsing into my chair, I ran a hand through my hair, grateful for my natural organization skills.

For months, Neil and I planned every detail of our wedding. We gathered brightly colored items to create a groovy theme. We incorporated vibrant blues, purples, oranges, and pinks into our decorations. We hand-picked upbeat music from the '60s and 70's to set the mood. Our buffet was filled with classic dishes like carved ham and roast while an open bar awaited our guests. Dress code? Tie-dye shirts and shorts - or anything groovy they wanted to wear. We were ready for the big day with everything checked off my to-do list and no last-minute surprises.

***

Internet Research:

Fatigue During Cancer Radiation Therapy (verywellhealth.com)

Fatigue occurs during radiation therapy because the body is working hard to repair the damage caused to healthy cells during treatment. The degree of fatigue generally varies depending on the amount of tissue irradiated, as well as the location.

***

Today's Quote:

"The more you lose yourself in something bigger than yourself, the more energy you will have."

—Norman Vincent Peale

A Note to You:

Being a bride just six days after your last round of treatment is not something I recommend. But with some serious backup, we pulled it off. Remember how you needed help during your cancer surgery? The same goes for radiation. As much as we want to be superheroes, we sometimes have to accept our human limitations. Take care of yourself first.

Cancer Post #41: Daughters Unite: June 16th

Ginger, my daughter, and Melissa, my bonus daughter, assisted me with the last-minute preparations. They collab-orated to create a magnificent bouquet of colorful ribbons and wildflowers. I beamed with joy at their creativity. After having lunch at a charming tea house, we went out for some retail therapy. Though I was feeling exhausted, the happy adrenaline rush kept me going. Unfortunately, my other bonus daughter Natalie couldn't join us due to work commitments. She offered to do my make-up for the wedding. Knowing her expertise in colors and shading, I felt confident I would look my best for the special occasion.

***

Internet Research:

Program Finder - Look Good Feel Better

The Look Good Feel Better group workshop provides hands-on makeup, skincare, wigs and head coverings techniques to help manage appearance-related side effects of cancer treatment. Women (age 18 or older) who are currently undergoing cancer treatment, about to undergo cancer treatment, or have recently completed cancer treatment (chemotherapy, radiation therapy, surgery, hormone therapy, or other forms of treatment) are eligible to attend.

***

Today's Quote:

"Each day comes bearing its own gifts. Untie the ribbons."

—Ruth Ann Schabacker

A Note to You:

There are days when we feel completely drained, and even brushing our teeth seems like a monumental task. But don't underestimate the power of trying to look good. Let yourself indulge in some new makeup or have a friend help you browse through online shops for a new wig or outfit. Remember, your beauty shines from within, and cancer can never take that away from you.

Cancer Post #42: Feeling Groovy: June 17th

The sun rose, signaling our wedding day. As I awoke, the strength of my bond with Neil flooded my mind, having weathered through life's trials. Grateful for such an extraordinary and awe-inspiring partner, I consciously tried to savor every moment we shared. No matter what the future held, he would always be my constant source of support and grounding.

The sound of laughter and conversation echoed in the house as relatives arrived one by one, embracing each other with cheerful hugs. I felt energized in the presence of so much love. I watched with wide-eyed enthusiasm as the girls and my new sister-in-law Kitty got to work decorating the ballroom for the wedding. They had pulled out all the stops to create a psychedelic wonderland, complete with an old VW cardboard hippie bus for photo ops.

As the afternoon dragged on, my energy waned. With the biggest evening of my life approaching, I realized I needed to recharge. Gratefully, everyone empathized as I departed the festivities and raced home for a quick power nap.

Neil and I arrived early to the event center, joining a sea of guests already swirling about with peace signs and headbands. Our tribe exuded wildness, clad in tie-dye shirts and hippie gear. The hotel guests must've been feeling groovy seeing around a hundred flower children, most of them in their sixties and seventies. Neil, my prince charming in his vibrant button-down shirt, groovy shorts, and tennis shoes, guided me through the crowd. My white sun dress from T.J. Maxx for twenty-four dollars was the epitome of bohemian chic. And perched atop my head was a veil made of pure white feathers.

My sister and I clasped hands, swinging them wildly in the air as we skipped down the aisle to the song "Feeling Groovy." It was time for the ceremony to begin! Linda, our old friend and minister, welcomed us with a warm smile before asking Neil if he would take me as his wedded wife. He responded without hesitation—with an enthusiastic "Groovy!" The guests erupted into laughter and cheers.

The night throbbed with music from the golden oldies, luring everyone onto the dance floor. Laughter reverberated off every wall. Beer bottles clinked, and wine glasses toasted in a joyous cacophony. Love was palpable as couples twirled to slow ballads. As the party came to an end, our DJ announced one last dance to the tune of "A

Groovy Kind of Love." Our young and old guests showered us with congratulations and declared our wedding the ultimate groovy celebration.

***

Internet Research:

A satisfying romantic relationship may improve breast cancer survivors' health ScienceDaily

Breast cancer survivors in romantic relationships who feel happy and satisfied with their partners may be at lower risk for a host of health problems, new research suggests.

***

Today's Quote:

"Being deeply loved by someone gives you strength, while loving someone deeply gives you courage."

—Lao Tzu

A Note to You:

Hey Pink Sisters, I'll admit I may sound like a lovesick teenager, but hear me out. Love transcends all boundaries - whether it's the bond between parents and children, friends, or even pets. It knows no gender nor sexual orientation. Every form of love is valid and beautiful.

Cancer Post #43: No Sex: June 17th

After bidding farewell to our loved ones, we shuffled into our hotel room. I was utterly drained, my body unable to handle any more physical exertion. While it is customary to consummate a marriage on the wedding night, I had no energy left. I asked my new husband if we could wait until our honeymoon started on Monday to be intimate. He said, "Sweetie, I'm exhausted, too."

   I knew I had chosen the right partner - someone who valued my need for rest over societal expectations.

***

Internet Research:

Regaining sexual health after cancer treatment - Mayo Clinic Comprehensive Cancer Center Blog

Sexual side effects from cancer treatment can cause added stress and anxiety, but they can be buffered by positive support from a partner, says Dr. Vencill. "It's important to have conversations around mental and emotional well-being, and to talk about sexual health when you feel ready."

***

Today's Quote:

"A sure sign of a man's strength is how gently he loves his wife."

—FierceMarriage.com

A Note to You:

For your husband to comprehend the interconnection between sex and breast cancer, direct him to the last chapter of this book, written by my husband. As we strive for mutual understanding in our relationships, let's not neglect nurturing empathy towards our loved ones. Go embrace your partner with a warm hug now.

NOTES AND THOUGHTS

CHAPTER TWELVE

MEN GET BREAST CANCER TOO

Cancer Post #44: Shadows of Breast Cancer: June 19th

Sunday morning dawned, and our extended family gathered for a final breakfast before departing from the wedding festivities. As everyone said their goodbyes, Neil's daughters stayed back a moment longer to give him warm embraces and heartfelt wishes for Father's Day. Watching this sweet exchange, it struck me that breast cancer affects men as well.

   The time has come to break the silence surrounding male breast cancer. While women are rightfully receiving attention and care for this deadly disease, men are being forgotten and are paying with their lives. Unbeknownst to many, nearly one percent of all diagnosed breast cancer cases worldwide are men. These men were not expecting to get what they considered a woman's disease.

***

Internet Research:

Male breast cancer – malecare.org

Both men and women are affected by breast cancer. However, the incidence is 100 times lesser in men. There is 1 in 1000 chances of a man developing breast cancer. This has remained unchanged for the last 30 years. In the US, nearly 2000 cases of breast cancer are reported in men. Men usually develop breast cancer in the later stages of life after 65 years of age.

General Information about Male Breast Cancer

- Male breast cancer is a disease in which malignant (cancer) cells form in the tissues of the breast.

- Radiation exposure, high levels of estrogen, and a family history of breast cancer can affect a man's risk of developing breast cancer.

- Male breast cancer is sometimes caused by inherited gene mutations (changes).

- Tests that examine the breasts are used to detect (find) and diagnose breast cancer in men.

- Survival for men with breast cancer is similar to survival for women with breast cancer.

- Certain factors affect prognosis (chance of recovery) and treatment options.

***

Today's Quote:

"Whether you're a mother or father, or a husband or a son, or a niece or a nephew or uncle, breast cancer doesn't discriminate."

—Stephanie McMahon

A Note to You:

Pink sisters, it's on us to spread the word about breast cancer affecting men, too. Don't shy away from talking to the men in your life about regularly checking for any abnormal lumps or bumps in their chest area. Let's make sure they know not to brush it off. We have the power to educate and raise awareness, so let's use it every chance we get.

SHELLEY MALICOTE STUTCHMAN

NOTES AND THOUGHTS

Chapter Thirteen
THE SHIFT

Cancer Post #45: Airport Security: June 20th

Our honeymoon was meant to be unforgettable, but not at the airport. Although my husband passed through security, the TSA lady barked at me, "Step over here," she demanded.

I stood frozen, hands in my pockets, unsure of what was happening. The security attendant locked eyes with me and barked, "You! Body search. Let's go."

The TSA officer firmly and meticulously patted down my left arm and underarm. Then quickly swept the rest of my body with precise efficiency. "You have been cleared," she declared.

I didn't fit the typical profiles of someone who would be pulled out of line - no suspicious behavior. Just an average old woman carrying a purse. Why did they single me out? Did they think I was hiding something? Or did they just need to meet their quota for random checks? Either way, it left me feeling bewildered and frustrated.

We boarded the plane to Austin. Neil and I clasped hands and exchanged loving smiles. His eyes twinkled mischievously when he teased me for being treated like a super spy. But our joy was uncontainable, for in Austin, Texas, awaited the beginning of our honeymoon and our life together as man and wife. We rented a car to take us to Fredericksburg and let love be our guide. Everywhere we went, hand in hand, we savored the exquisite wines, indulged in delectable cuisine, and embraced each other in passionate kisses.

After five glorious days, we were back at the airport. Neil sailed through the airport security. But then, just like before, the TSA guard's command sliced through the air: "Step aside!"

How could this be happening again?

The security officer looked me up and down with suspicion and then instructed me to remove my compression sleeve. My lymphatic therapist warned me that the air pressure in the cabin could cause swelling if I didn't wear it. The realization struck me like a lightning bolt - was this why I'd been pulled aside in Oklahoma City? Before she could answer, I explained why I was wearing the sleeve and why. She nodded knowingly — apparently, people had worn them before and used them to sneak items onto planes that they weren't allowed to have.

I wore my sleeve on the plane. However, when I arrived home, my arm was fine, but my left breast had swelled up like a balloon. Breast lymphedema occurs because of damage to the lymphatic system. I am guessing that the lymphedema in my breast may have happened because I flew only ten days after my last radiation treatment. I looked like one of the Kardashians on my left and an ordinary woman on my right. I hoped it would reduce in size before I returned to work. Anyway, for my new husband, I looked like a centerfold from the left and a librarian from the right—nothing like variety, they say.

***

Internet Research:

How to Plan for Air Travel with Lymphedema - Flow Lymphatic Health Clinic

Planning a trip is exciting to think about. However, air travel may affect your lymphedema or trigger the onset. Not everyone is affected by air travel and there is research* to show this. In clinical practice we have seen enough patients who are affected so it's worth noting and taking simple precautions.

When we fly our tissues are affected by the cabin pressure. Our tissue pressure is normally a negative value; it has a suction effect as it pulls inward to keep our tissue tight against blood and lymph vessels. When tissue pressure weakens, it can cause more fluid to enter the tissues from the blood vessels than normal, and at the same time is weak to push fluid into the lymphatics and shows up as swelling. When we fly, the altitude changes our tissue pressure to move toward the direction of positive. Tissue pressure becomes weaker and may result in more fluid accumulating in the tissues because the force to keep fluid in the blood vessels has weakened.

Compression garments act to replace lost or weakened tissue pressure. If you have lymphedema, it would be advised to wear your compression garment before, during, and after a flight.

***

Today's Quote:

"Toughness is in the soul and spirit, not in muscles."

—Alex Karras

A Note to You:

My dear sister, we've been through so much together, and sometimes, strangers have the most unexpected reactions. But instead of letting their uneducated and idiotic remarks stress us out, let's find the humor in it all. It'll save us a lot of unnecessary worry and frustration.

Cancer Post #46: Shifting Priorities: June 24th

During our honeymoon, I pondered and meditated. Sitting on the serene patio of our cottage, overlooking the babbling river with graceful deer drinking the cool water, I connected with my innermost self. In my pocket notebook, I scribbled down my musings. I refused to let go of the thoughts dancing through my mind as I underwent a spiritual awakening. It was a moment of pure tranquility, rejuvenating my soul's purpose.

The cancer diagnosis shattered my illusions of immortality, forcing me to contemplate life in a new light. My priorities shifted drastically as I embraced a deeper understanding of the universe and my place in it. Each person's transformation is unique, but I will endeavor to articulate mine here.

1. Choose what God wants me to do today:

With the first rays of dawn, I will commune with the Divine and inquire, "What is your purpose for me today?" I must not waste my fleeting moments on this Earth.

2. The Core of Who I Am:

For many years, my main focus was on gaining acceptance and validation from others. Society often told me that being a people-pleaser was wrong, an unattainable standard to chase after. However, my perspective shifted when I battled cancer. It helped me understand and appreciate my true nature: a person who finds joy in making others smile. Being a people-pleaser is not about seeking approval, but finding fulfillment in bringing happiness to those around me.

3. Don't Fear Change:

Cancer has been a harsh teacher, but has also shown me the power of change. One positive test result was all it took to shift my entire perspective. I used to fear the unknown, the challenges that lay ahead. But now, I'm calm. I have found strength within myself to face anything that comes my way. Cancer has given me resilience and taught me that I can conquer any changes in life on my own; I have become my own superhero. I may not be a Superwoman, but I am one strong and capable woman.

4. Don't Self Deprecate:

Every time I stared at my mirror reflection, I harshly criticized myself. "You're too heavy. You're aging rapidly. Your eyes appear exhausted. Your hair lacks luster. Your skin is losing its elasticity."

I often fell for the lure of buying the newest and most fantastic product, convinced that it would give me back my youth. Sometimes, it did have a negligible effect. But despite my hopes, the reflection staring back at me from the glossy surface was far from the thirty-five-year-old I envisioned in my mind.

Years of striving for perfection have been replaced by gazing at myself with compassion. After my battle with cancer, I now greet my reflection with a smile, affirming, "Great work, Shelley, you're alive! Now go out into the world and bask in the beauty of the day."

5. Don't Live in the Past:

I often ruminated on choices I've regretfully made, lamenting that I couldn't go back in time to change them. My battle with cancer taught me that life moves forward, never backward. There was no rewind. I frequently grappled with the desire to reverse some of the bad decisions I made in life, yet I've learned this was impossible. What's left was to focus on the here and now, savoring each moment and making the most of it by doing good.

6. Don't Let Anything Define Me:

Self-reliance was a source of pride for me, even though it could be difficult for those who cared about me. Cancer taught me the importance of staying true to myself and not letting anyone else's opinions shape me. I refused to let my age, any illness, outside perceptions, or physical appearance define who I am. You might wonder how I could value independence yet still be a people-pleaser; it may seem contradictory, but the balance of being self-sufficient and welcoming made me who I am.

7. Drama:

While fighting cancer, I couldn't handle any additional stress. I asked my loved ones to shield me from unnecessary drama. Cancer required all my energy and attention to heal, and I had to block out any external distractions. Before my battle with cancer, I wouldn't have had the courage to express my needs to others. This experience taught me the importance of standing up for myself and not allowing others to take advantage of me. I learned I can't heal or come up with a solution to other people's drama. I can have a sympathetic ear, but I can no longer try to solve their struggles. Cancer taught me that just as no one could make what I was going through disappear, I couldn't do that for others either. I can give a hug, a text of encouragement, or one of the millions of things people did for me to ease the crisis, but I don't have the power to solve the problems of others. I realized after all these years the people going through their drama must find their solutions and peace. I vow to no longer try to fix the world.

8. Spiritual:

My faith faltered. Why did God give me cancer? The stock market kept plummeting. Basic necessities became unaffordable for many. School shootings plagued our nation. Political divisions tore us apart. I pleaded for my son's healing, but it seemed like God remained indifferent. "Does He even care?" I wondered.

Then it hit me like a ton of bricks – I didn't want to argue with God anymore. I wanted to find my faith again, like when I was a child: trust more, worry less. So many people prayed for me, and I was alive, living in a brand-new house, and married to a good man. My son's illness seemed under control. Sitting on the porch one night after we were back from our honeymoon, I said to God, "If you care, show me by sending a hummingbird to this feeder."

Two hummingbirds showed up almost immediately. It felt like an answer from God, and everything suddenly made sense. It became clear that we have free will; our responsibility is to be the best people we can be. What happens after that is out of our control. I committed to keeping my faith alive, and when I finally get to heaven, then I'll understand the questions beyond my earthly comprehension.

9. Useful Purpose:

Since my cancer diagnosis, I've realized it's not prudent to be irked by the mundane trials of life. The traffic didn't go faster if I was angry because someone was slowing down the pacing; no good would come from lashing out at someone's remark, and robocalls wouldn't cease if I seethed with frustration. Instead, I chose to focus my energies on positive thoughts that would lift me up and help me live a useful and purposeful life.

10. Peace:

There are two people I know who radiate an aura of serenity. In their company, I feel tranquility. They inspired me to embody that same energy. Through diligent effort and conscious intention, my ultimate aspiration was to exude peace wherever I roam.

11. Someday:

Someday never comes. So often, I'm guilty of making plans and saying, "Someday, let's have lunch. Someday, let's take in a movie. Someday, let's do this or that."

But I recognize that "some days" don't count. If I wanted to make something happen, I set a date and turn it into reality. There was no room left for procrastination or pushing things off to a distant tomorrow.

12. Cancer Club:

Cancer creates an ineffable connection between us. When I meet another who has been through the same fight, a sense of solidarity immediately reverberates throughout our souls. As a cancer survivor, I promise to pay it forward and be a helping hand to those just beginning their journey.

13. Like equates Like:

When I was in college, one of my professors said, "Like equates like."

He explained, "When you meet people, instantly like them. They will like you back."

Cancer reminds me of that lesson. I plan to put it into constant practice. I may even blurt out to someone, "Hey, I like you."

14. Superpower:

I'm pretty sure I've gained a superpower from all that radiation. I am still determining what it is, but I'm hoping it involves being able to turn pizza into money. Crossing my fingers for the next time I order a large pepperoni.

***

Internet Research:

New Meanings and Shifting Priorities (survivingbreastcancer.org)

If you want to know what's most important in life, just ask a woman who's been diagnosed with breast cancer. Facing her mortality makes the little things fall away, and the big things come into laser-sharp focus.

***

Today's Quote:

"I am not this hair, I am not this skin, I am the soul that lives within."

—Rumi

A Note to You:

My pink sister, go to a peaceful place and bring your pens and journals. Write about all the growth and shifts you've gone through with cancer. If you're feeling inspired, take on the fourteen subjects I ruminated on and write down your insights. But don't just stash these away - read them repeatedly until you're living them out loud. This kind of introspection is medicine for your soul.

PEEK-A-BOOB

NOTES AND THOUGHTS

Chapter Fourteen

CHAINED

Cancer Post #47: Revving Up: June 26th

I penned a long and rambling email the night before returning to work, warning my team that transitioning back to my everyday workload might be difficult. I offered detailed explanations of why I had been away so long, how it had changed me, and how the expectations my job required would be different from my usual production for a while. Below is the email I sent to colleagues.

Hello, Team,

I am looking forward to seeing all of you again. Since June 1st, it has been quite a ride.

I wanted to ensure you knew that I have quite a few more medical visits scheduled. The next few months are crucial in the efforts to prevent the Big C from coming back.

The doctors are optimistic that the radiation therapy successfully eliminated all my cancer cells. They estimated that there is only a 3% chance of it returning. Starting on Friday, I will begin taking medication to further reduce my risk. However, there is a potential for serious side effects from the drug. I hope everything will go smoothly and I won't experience any issues. Below is detailed information about my cancer so you can have a better idea of where I am at in the world of this disease.

Here is my data:

Percentage of Cells with Nuclear Positivity: 100%

The nuclear grade describes how closely the nuclei of cancer cells look like the nuclei of normal breast cells. In general, the higher the nuclear grade, the more abnormal the nuclei are, and the more aggressive the tumor cells tend to be.

More Data:

Ki-67 Percentage of Positive Nuclei: 20 %

In the test results, you will see the Ki-67 findings expressed as a percentage. This is the percentage of the total sample that has active Ki-67 proteins. This is used to estimate how many cells are actively dividing, as follows:

Less than 10% is considered low.

20% or higher is considered high.

A high percentage means that the breast tumor is more likely to be aggressive and spread quickly.

I was fortunate to discover the tumor early and had it expertly removed. Just a month or two of delays could have meant chemotherapy. The doctors are optimistic about my odds of survival. Still, I must be vigilant and monitor myself carefully for any sign of a recurrence.

***

Internet Research:

Returning to Work After Breast Cancer Treatment: Ways to Make the Transition Smoother

Schedule a return-to-work meeting with any people you work with, including your supervisor and colleagues. Having a meeting when you return is a good opportunity to let everyone know you're ready to resume your responsibilities, especially if you had to reduce your hours or hand off projects to others. It's also a good opportunity to let everyone know whether or not you prefer to avoid discussions about breast cancer.

There are protections in place to help you. The Americans with Disabilities Act (ADA) requires employers to provide reasonable accommodations for people with physical limitations because of medical conditions. The ADA applies to private businesses and organizations as well as government employers. Examples include flexible scheduling, time off for appointments, reassignment to a more suitable position, adjustments in the workspace, and modifications to equipment and technology. The Job Accommodation Network is a great starting point for more information about your rights.

***

Today's Quote:

"Cancer is a word, not a sentence."

—John Diamond

A Note to You:

When you return to work, remember that taking things slow and not feeling pressured to be as efficient and precise as before is okay. Your team will understand if you communicate with them about your current state of healing and how it may affect your productivity. Each workplace has its own unique culture, so it's important to adapt and decide how much information you want to share with your colleagues regarding your battle with cancer. It's also important not to compare yourself to others who may have returned to work sooner after treatment; we all have our own pace in recovery. Just do what feels right for you - there is no right or wrong way in this situation.

Cancer Post #48: Chained: June 27th

When I walked through the doors of my workplace, the familiar hum of computers and chatter hit my ears like a wave. I had been absent for nearly a month, but it felt like years. In that brief time frame, I had undergone brachytherapy, married my soul mate, and ventured off on a romantic honeymoon. It was dizzying to think about everything that had transpired in such a short amount of time. I stepped into the office, ready to take on whatever awaited me.

A part of me felt chained to my disease. I worried about taking any days off work, even for a vacation, because what if there was a recurrence and I needed to save my paid time off for that? The potential side effects of the new medicine I would soon start weighed heavily on my mind. And could I really trust that the reconstruction surgery scheduled for November would go smoothly? What if my energy levels never returned to normal? These constant "what ifs" left me feeling powerless. I desperately needed to break free from Cancer's chain, or I would be forever entrapped in a world of missed opportunities and wasted life.

***

Internet Research:

6 Ways to Stop Worrying About Your Cancer Returning and Live Your Life curetoday.com)

Rather than worry about the future none of us can control, focus on taking care of yourself, accepting your cancer may come back, embracing your worry and fears by writing about them, having a talk with yourself, meditating, praying, or both, and then living the best life you can.

***

Today's Quote:

"Hope is like the sun, which, as we journey toward it, casts the shadow of our burden behind us."

—Samuel Smiles

A Note to You:

Next time the What Ifs come knocking at your door, have a little conversation with yourself. It could go something like this:

Your Mind: "I'm afraid my cancer will return."

You: "Why worry about something you can't control?"

Your Mind: "It makes me feel like I'm doing something."

You: "There are better things to spend your time on than worrying about a potential future event."

Your Mind: "But I'm still scared."

You: "If fear is consuming you, channel that energy towards something productive. Don't waste your valuable time listening to your Mind's attempts to unsettle you."

Cancer Post #49: My Second Day Back to Work: June 28th

On my second day back to work, I was already crisscrossing the city, driving from my office on one side of town to my lymphedema appointment at 9 AM, then the opposite part of the city to the radiologist by lunchtime. I was glad I had forewarned my team of these medical appointments.

My lymphedema therapist sat on the edge of my bed and adjusted her glasses as she studied me. She took a deep breath before shaking her head and softly said, "You set up the perfect storm for your lymphedema."

She explained that flying only ten days after radiation had triggered my breast to swell again. It hurt and felt heavy. I couldn't help but immediately think it must be a cancer recurrence. She calmed me down assuring me it was inflammation and swelling, and then spent an hour kneading my chest with lymphatic drainage massage techniques to reduce the severity of the condition. While it was a strange experience to have someone massage my breast for so long, her magic hands worked wonders as the balloon-like shape disappeared, and the pain subsided.

After my therapy appointment, I returned to work for an hour before heading to the radiologist. Upon arrival, I was relieved to see her appointments running on time since I needed to return to work. I asked her to feel my breast, searching for any lumps that may have developed since my last appointment.

I thought about the rash that had slowly spread across my chest over the past few days—it itched like crazy—and wondered if I'd been a fool not to realize it could be Inflammatory Breast Cancer. When I asked about it, she gently assured me it was merely a rash caused by radiation exposure and prescribed a steroid pack.

I struggled to stay within my desired weight, so I decided not to take the steroids. Instead, I used a topical ointment for my rash. My scale would swing five pounds in three days. I was doing everything right: eating healthy foods and exercising regularly. I couldn't understand why I was having such difficulty. What the heck was going on?

***

Internet Research:

Inflammatory Breast Cancer: Signs, Symptoms, Causes & Treatment clevelandclinic.org)

Inflammatory breast cancer is a rare, fast-growing cancer that requires immediate treatment. It causes symptoms similar to a breast infection. Signs of IBC may include redness, swelling, pain, enlargement of one breast and breast skin that resembles an orange peel. Treatments include chemotherapy, surgery and radiation.

***

Today's Quote:

"Fear defeats more people than any other thing in the world."

—Ralph Waldo Emerson

A Note to You:

Let me give you some advice about balancing doctor appointments and work. Always tell your boss you'll be gone an extra hour than you actually think it'll take. If the doctor is running behind or your appointment takes longer than expected, you're covered. And if things go smoothly and you're out earlier than planned, you'll earn brownie points for returning early. It's all about turning a potentially stressful situation into a win-win for yourself.

NOTES AND THOUGHTS

CHAPTER FIFTEEN

HORMONE HORROR

Cancer Post #50:
To Letrozole or Not to Letrozole:
June 30th

I struggled with the choice of whether or not to take Letrozole. On the one hand, my oncologist seemed confident it would help prevent a recurrence. On the other, I felt hesitant because of the potential side effects. Her suggestion I wait until I was back from my honeymoon seemed so considerate on the surface. However, this suggestion only heightened my fear the medicine could be nasty if she didn't want it to interfere with my honeymoon. What should I do?

I turned to Dr. Google.

The first statement on the Letrozole page showed a woman with a bubble over her head and a questioning look. In the bubble, this sentence materialized, "Anti-estrogen therapy is not fun. But nothing is worse than the fear of my cancer coming back."

At the following P31 Breast Cancer Support Group, ladies shared their experiences with hormone blockers. One woman rubbed her stiff fingers together, wincing as she did so. Another smoothed her thinning hair. "I had no idea everything could get so dry," another said, pointing to her southern lady parts.

Weight gain seemed to be universal among these women. Our struggles bound us together, but seeing so much pain from this medication scared me.

Another lady pleaded with me to take the pill. A bright purple scarf covered her bald head, and I heard the sound of regret in her voice, "I stopped taking it because of the side effects," she said softly. "But then my cancer came back. My doctor said it probably wouldn't have happened if I had just stayed on the medication."

The conversation with her made me reevaluate my opinion. I wavered, thinking maybe I should at least try the medication. I knew I could always quit if anything went wrong.

Another lady relayed a vivid description of the kind of dryness the pill causes. "It makes your hoo-ha feel like crepe paper, honey!"

As a newlywed, I imagined my intimate area covered in thin layers of crispy tissue paper and shuddered. The joint pain, weight gain, and undesirable side effects worried me, so I wavered again, choosing perhaps not taking it. I needed to make a firm decision. I was driving myself crazy, going back and forth on this issue.

When I got home after the meeting, I sat with my hands on my lap, studying the list of Letrozole's side effects scrawled across a piece of paper. None of them appealed to me. I thought back to when I was younger and vigorous and could have handled any obstacle that came my way. Now, in my late sixties, I only wanted to enjoy life for as long as possible.

I scrolled through the thousands of reviews on Dr. Google about Letrozole, skimming to get a sense of the overall sentiment. Here is a sample of things I read repeatedly from the reviews:

- Severe back pain.
- Severe hip pain.
- Severe knee pain.
- Muscle fatigue.
- Sleepless nights.
- Feeling exhausted all the time.
- No quality of life.
- Worse than chemotherapy.
- Hair loss.
- Cognitive decline.
- Loss of libido.
- Feeling like I'm ninety years old.
- Hot flashes.
- Weight gain.
- Blurry vision.

The next morning, I looked at that yellow pill; I could flush the Letrozole prescription down the toilet or decide to try it. The fear of cancer recurring won out. I brought the capsule to my mouth and forced myself to swallow it. A short prayer escaped my lips, "God, please make this medicine work and protect me from its side effects. Amen."

I approached my colleagues at work, requesting their vigilant observation of any changes in my behavior while taking this medication. I feared becoming a negative and difficult-to-work-with individual. However, the first day of taking the medication proceeded smoothly without any adverse effects.

That evening, I got on my P31 Facebook support page. I clicked through to the comment thread of women on this drug. Many suggested taking Claritin daily with the pill. They said it helped lessen their joint pain. Some of the ladies added that they couldn't get their doctors to agree, but for them, it worked. I went to my Amazon page and ordered Claritin that night.

I closed my eyes and took a deep breath. I thought about the words drilled into my mind since childhood. "Your thoughts shape your reality."

For this to work, I had to keep my chin up and look at it from the right angle. I had to believe that taking this medicine could reduce my risk of reoccurrence.

The following morning, I rolled the medicine bottle around in my hand and read the warning label once again.

Warnings:

You should not use letrozole if you are pregnant.

Well, that was my first positive to start the day. Thank goodness I wasn't pregnant at age sixty-seven, although it would have been quite a feat if I had managed it!

I decided to give the pill a shot for one week, and then I would reevaluate my decision.

***

Internet Research:

Letrozole: How It Works & Side Effects (clevelandclinic.org)

LETROZOLE (LET roe zole) treats some types of breast cancer. It works by decreasing the amount of estrogen hormone your body makes, which slows or stops breast cancer cells from spreading or growing.

***

Today's Quote:

"A generation ago breast cancer was a dreaded disease spoken about in hushed tones by our mothers…The survival rate was only 50% and mastectomy was inevitable. The story couldn't be more different today. Survival rates are soaring and treatment by lumpectomy or with reconstruction means avoiding disfigurement….I believe that breast cancer will soon become something we live with rather than die from."

—Lindsay Nicholson, Good Housekeeping Editor and Breast Cancer Survivor

A Note to You:

If your doctors bring up a hormone blocker, make sure to do your own research and don't be afraid to ask them for the truth about your risk of recurrence with or without it. Your health is too important to just trust blindly.

Cancer Post #51: Hilarious Hazards of Cancer: July 1st

No matter how dire your circumstances are, a spark of humor can usually be found. Amidst the pain and suffering of cancer, you must search for moments to laugh to keep you going.

As I navigated the car through the streets on our way to lunch, a solemn thought crossed my mind. "I'm worried about dying from cancer," I said quietly to my friend.

My friend said, "That's not a problem."

Surprised, I remarked, "It's not?"

She answered, "You are more likely to die in a car crash."

I asked, "Why do you say that?"

She said, "Let's just say, I'm your passenger, and I am praying right now that we make it to our lunch destination alive."

I laughed so hard I thought I might wreck the car.

***

Internet Research:

The power of laughter for cancer patients (cancercenter.com)

Sometimes, allowing yourself the time, and room, to see the humor in some of life's lighter moments can bring levity to the situation. In those moments, choosing to laugh is like a booster shot to your resilience, with no unpleasant side effects and hopefully some unexpectedly pleasant ones.

Although laughter may seem like an uncontrolled reaction to something funny, scientists have determined that our bodies can't really tell the difference between authentic laughter and a process behavioral health therapists like to call, "Fake it 'til you make it!" The simple act of laughing can be strong enough to take over your body, and can lead to chemical changes that can actually shift your perspective, even if you're not reacting to something funny but laughing just to laugh.

***

Today's Quote:

"How many cancer patients does it take to screw in a light bulb? Just one, but they have a big support group cheering them on. We're all here for you!"

—Anonymous

A Note for You:

No matter what kind of day you're having, give yourself a break and enjoy a funny video. And believe it or not, there are even jokes about cancer on the internet! It may seem twisted, but if that type of humor appeals to you, you should check them out. Humor has the power to turn your day around for the better.

Cancer Post #52: Thrills and Chills Hormone Horrors: July 8th

What a ride the past seven days were. When your hormones are out of balance, all I can say is, "You are in for a bumpy ride, cowgirl."

I ingested those pills on Friday, July 1st, with the hope that nothing would occur. As the weekend and the following week passed, my concerns diminished. I couldn't believe my luck; no single side effect from the medication appeared. With a deep sigh of relief, I celebrated my good fortune.

Wednesday at midnight I felt the sudden onset of pain. My joints in my knees, hips, and legs burned ferociously, making it impossible to stay asleep. I decided not to take painkillers since I had to work the following morning. Instead, I opted to stay up and distract myself. I climbed the stairs to my home office. I spent a few hours mindlessly scrolling through Facebook and doing computer-related tasks. The discomfort had disappeared by three in the morning, so I returned to bed.

On Thursday morning, I hesitated but took another Letrozole. During our daily huddle at work, I asked our chaplain to pray I wouldn't experience any more side effects from the medication. That night, when I rested my head on my pillow, I slept like a baby—no joint pain nor other side effects. The following Friday, I woke up feeling grateful for this miracle.

After one week of taking the medication, I experienced minor joint pain, but tolerable. However, I couldn't help but worry about the severe drop in my energy levels. While most newlyweds were busy building their new life together, I found myself exhausted by 8 pm every night, unable to do anything but slump on the couch and watch TV until bedtime. I lacked the energy to even make a dent in my to-do list. I used to be able to power through my exhaustion and keep going. But with this pill, it was different; once the fatigue set in, the couch became my closest companion.

Friday evening, Neil took me to a swanky restaurant for dinner, and our conversation flowed. But, on the journey home, tears rolled down my cheeks, yet I didn't know why. The entire fiasco left me wrung out. I collapsed onto the couch to watch some mindless TV. Unfortunately, I had duties as the Saturday manager at work that demanded I be up early the following morning. I retired to bed around ten on Friday night. While lying in bed an onslaught of tears turned into sorrowful sobs; my desire for living was at its most brittle ebb. In my mind's eye, I deeply contemplated oblivion by taking a bottle of pills and finally being free from this cancer-ridden life and all the crap that came with cancer.

Though I didn't really want to act on them, thoughts of ending my life kept entering my mind. Unable to find sleep, I picked up my phone in the wee hours of the morning. I scrolled to my P31 cancer support Facebook page and asked why this sudden depression had struck me and why these suicidal notions crept in.

The responses flooded in. Several people wrote they experienced the same feelings. Since this medicine blocks estrogen production, hormones become way off balance. Most people said to give it a little time and that things would stabilize. One lady wrote, "The first month on Letrozole is hell. Then you return to your happy self."

I lay awake in bed, my mind heavy with dread as I pondered if the blues would still linger when I awoke. But, much to my relief, they had dissipated.

At work, I chatted with some of the residents who were breast cancer survivors. They spoke of their struggles adjusting to hormone-blocking drugs. The women embraced me with supportive hugs and gentle words of encouragement. My mood brightened, and I even managed a few laughs amidst our conversation.

I returned home from work feeling uplifted. That night, I cherished every moment spent bonding with my husband until a surprising hour - eleven o'clock! - before drifting into a peaceful sleep. What a rollercoaster of emotions those twenty-four hours had been.

At first, it seemed like an easy choice. When I started taking this pill, I said I would quit if I felt any side effects. But as the days went by, my conviction faltered. I watched YouTube videos on Letrozole and saw the potential for preventing cancer from coming back. The thought of facing this disease for a second time terrified me.

On the other hand, this drug could cause serious health risks that I wasn't sure I was ready to take. Every day, I again found myself struggling with this decision. In the end, I decided to continue trying it a bit longer. I wanted to live.

I wish the doctors who prescribe this medication would tell us the truth about the side effects we might experience. Instead, all they do is shrug and say, "Every person reacts differently." As if that will make us feel any better!

***

Internet Research:

Hormonal imbalance and depression: What to know (medicalnewstoday.com)

A drop in hormones can lead to a reduced level of serotonin, which can result in increased levels of sadness, anxiety, and irritability. Hormonal changes may cause depression in some people.

***

Today's Quote:

"No matter what happens, or how bad it seems today, life does go on, and it will be better tomorrow."

—Maya Angelou

A Note to You:

As I delved deeper into my research and conversed with the members of my breast cancer support group, P31, I felt a sense of sisterhood. We have all been on this tumultuous journey together, and understanding each other's struggles has brought us closer. So, if you're struggling with mood swings from this medication, know that you are not alone. Many of us have experienced similar side effects and can offer solace and support. There truly is strength in numbers, especially among women fighting against breast cancer.

NOTES AND THOUGHTS

CHAPTER SIXTEEN

CELEBRATE

Cancer Post #53: One Month Cancer Free: July 10th

June 10th represented my final day of brachytherapy. Neil and I both reached out for the rope coiled around the bell, pulling it together. As the bell clanged loudly above us, Neil smiled and said, "From now on, we'll celebrate every tenth day of the month as one more month free from cancer."

On July 10th, we went to our favorite spot, Pub W, to celebrate and enjoy the moment! Jill, our bartender, snapped a picture of our celebration. In recognition of this milestone, she presented me with a complimentary mimosa. It truly felt like a victory, like I had crossed the finish line.

I savored every bite of my Nutella Belgian waffle, knowing it was an indulgence that wasn't exactly healthy. Despite this, I decided to make the 10th day of each month a day to eat whatever my heart desired without any guilt or restrictions.

I'm grateful for my husband's heartwarming gesture of making the tenth of each month a special day to remember. His desire to create beautiful memories is truly admirable, showing how much, he values and loves me. I'm so thankful for his kindness and for making the world a better place for me, one special day at a time.

***

Internet Research:

https://www.mycancerchic.com/ways-to-celebrate-being-cancer-free

Ten ways to celebrate being cancer-free:

- Have a special photoshoot.

- Plan for the future.

- Go on a physical outing.

- Celebrate with loved ones.

- Pamper yourself.

- Give back to the cancer community

- Plan a vacation.

- Get a tattoo.

- Get a haircut.

- Buy a body-friendly outfit.

***

Today's Quote:

"My cancer scare changed my life. I'm grateful for every new, healthy day I have. It has helped me prioritize my life."

—Olivia Newton-John

A Note to You:

When you finally get to ring that bell, pause and reflect on your arduous battle with cancer. Celebrate this momentous achievement and recognize when you felt like giving up but pushed through and came out victorious. You did it! And now, every month, take a day to commemorate your strength and resilience. Indulge in your favorite meal, take a break from work to do something you enjoy, or spend quality time with those who stood by you throughout your journey. You deserve it, my dear friend.

# NOTES AND THOUGHTS

CHAPTER SEVENTEEN

THE FINE LINE BETWEEN PARANOID AND CAUTIOUS

Cancer Post #54: Invisible Intruders: July 17th

On Sunday, I felt a throbbing pain in my head, achy muscles, nausea, fatigue, and shivers. Monday, it was like I had been mowed down by a Mac Truck. My fever peaked at 103 degrees, and it seemed like whatever virus had attacked me was taking advantage of the situation.

I called my boss to let her know I wouldn't be in to work. Cathy urged me to check for COVID with an at-home test. My sister chimed in her agreement; worry laced through her words. The rest of my family sent texts and messages. I thought I had the flu. It was just a temporary setback that would be over in twenty-four to forty-eight hours. Besides, my primary care doctor was on vacation. What good would it do to call?

But my boss and sister persisted, their concern palpable even through the digital connection. With a sigh, I called my oncologist's nurse. She told me many things were going around, to take Motrin followed by Tylenol every three or four hours.

Neil and I didn't have any Covid test kits. Our friend Bill offered to give us his. Neil picked up the test and brought it home. Even though I wanted to take it, I was unsure how to follow the instructions because my head was pounding, and I couldn't concentrate. Neil took over and administered the test. Thankfully, the results came back negative.

My boss and sister explained to me that life would be different while living with cancer. They both told me I couldn't blow off a virus like I used to. This piece of information is something none of my cancer doctors shared with me. Even if my doctors omitted the details, I had people around me who could help me understand. There were far too many unknowns and uncertainties to count.

After hearing from my boss and sister, I checked The American Cancer Society website. They were correct. I couldn't help but feel frustrated that my team of five doctors didn't inform me not to blow off something I thought could be a virus.

I woke up in the middle of the night, drenched in sweat, and my sheets were damp. Surprisingly, this was a good sign. As the hours passed, I felt better and was able to return to work the next day.

***

Internet Research:

Risk for Infection and Cancer (verywellhealth.com)

Being diagnosed with cancer has likely been one of the most stressful periods of your life. This is an overwhelming time, and having to worry about further complications like the risk of infection may feel like too much. Know that your body is not as capable of fighting off infections right now, so it is essential to monitor yourself for any signs, such as a fever. Talk with your healthcare provider about how to protect yourself from infection.

***

Today's Quote:

"Love and laughter are two of the most important universal cancer treatments on the planet. Overdose on them."

—Tanya Masse

A Note to You:

I know the doctors may not tell you this, but you need to be on high alert. With all those cancer treatments, your immune system is compromised, and you're at a higher risk of catching any bug that's going around. So, don't forget to use hand sanitizer as if it's your full-time job, okay?

Cancer Post #55: Sick Again: July 25th

To my surprise, I fell ill once again within a week of recovering from my last virus. As someone who rarely got sick, this was not my usual experience. When my symptoms became more severe, I decided to go to the emergency room for medical care. My temperature had risen to 104 degrees. The doctor performed a quick COVID test and tests for Influenzas A & B, but all results returned negative.

The doctor gave me a prescription for Tylenol and an IV drip to reduce my temperature and keep me hydrated. "So, if I'm not infected with Covid or the flu, why am I experiencing a high fever, chills, headaches, and body aches?" I inquired.

She studied me carefully, but the cause of my symptoms remained a mystery. I asked her if my breast could have an infection since it felt so swollen and heavy. She nodded as she considered the possibility, then told me I should call my surgeon in the morning. Even though she had given me a possible answer, I still didn't know for sure.

I struggled to understand the source of my illness. Suddenly, it hit me - the lessons I had learned during my battle with cancer echoed in my mind: be your own doctor, do your own research. While still in the E.R., I turned to Dr. Google for answers.

First, I decided to check if the cancer pill Letrozole I am on can cause flu-like symptoms. Here is what I found on Drugs.com

Check with your doctor immediately if any of the following side effects occur while taking letrozole:
Less common
- Bone fracture
- breast pain
- chest pain
- chills, fever, or flu-like symptoms
- mental depression
- swelling of the feet or lower legs

After leaving the ER, I still didn't have any answers. I decided to take matters into my own hands and closely examine the lab results made available to me on my portal. Scrutinizing the details, I discovered the root of the issue - something that the ER doctor had failed to identify. I couldn't help but feel frustrated the doctor had overlooked such a crucial piece of information.

LYMPHOCYTES

Mine 9%   Normal: 24% to 44%

Unusually high or low lymphocyte counts may cause no signs, symptoms, or serious problems on their own. They can be the body's normal response to an infection, inflammatory condition, or other unusual condition and will return to normal levels after some time.

Lymphocytes are white blood cells and one of the body's main types of immune cells. They are made in the bone marrow and found in the blood and lymph tissue.

Lymphocytes getting stuck in the lymph nodes is one of the reasons for the low number.

The Glucose levels surprised me. I rarely eat sweets or fried foods. Yet my level was 130 mg, and normal is 90 to 110 mg.

Glucose levels can be normal, high, or low, depending on how much glucose someone has in their bloodstream. Glucose is a basic sugar that is available in the bloodstream consistently. Normal blood glucose levels can be estimated when someone diets, eats, or after they've eaten. A normal blood glucose level for grown-ups without diabetes who haven't eaten for at least eight hours (fasting) is under 100 mg/dL. A normal blood glucose level for adults without diabetes two hours after eating is 90 to 110 mg/d

I wondered, am I pre-diabetic?

Leukocyte esterase is a urine test to look for white blood cells and other signs of infection

My Result 1+

Standard Result is negative.

This result made me wonder if I had a possible UTI.

KETONES UA

My Result 2+

Normal Result is negative

Our body typically uses glucose, or sugar, as the main source of energy. When cells don't get the glucose they need, the body begins to use fat instead. Burning fat produces ketones, a type of acid that ends up in your blood and urine that can make you very sick.

If you feel very unwell or a urine ketone test result is more than 2+, then there's a high chance you have DKA, requiring emergency medical care and treatment in a hospital immediately.

Since I was 2+, I felt unwell; why was nothing done? Oh, so many questions I had.

BILIRUBIN UA

My Result 1+

Normal Result is negative

Bilirubin in urine test measures the levels of bilirubin in your urine. Normally, urine doesn't have any bilirubin. If there is bilirubin in your urine, it may be an early sign of a liver condition.

Bilirubin is a yellow substance your body makes during the normal process of breaking down red blood cells. Your liver uses bilirubin to make bile, a fluid that helps you digest food.

A healthy liver removes most of the bilirubin from your body. But if there is a problem with your liver, bilirubin can build up in your blood and get into your urine.

The liver is one of the places breast cancer spreads—another question for the doctors.

Blood UA

My Result 2+

Normal Result is Negative

Urinary occult blood 2+ needs treatment. In normal urine routine results, urine occult blood should be negative. If the examination finds urine occult blood 2+, it indicates the presence of red blood cells in the urine, leading to a positive result. Urinary occult blood is caused mainly by nephritis, cystitis, other urinary system infections, bladder stones, kidney stones, and urethral stones. The cause should be found in time, and the corresponding drug treatment should be selected according to the reason.

WBC UA

My Result 6-10 /hpf

Normal Result 0 - 2 /hpf

WBC stands for White Blood Cells

Urine is generally thought of as a sterile body fluid. Therefore, evidence of white blood cells or bacteria in the urine is considered abnormal and may suggest a urinary tract infection such as bladder infection (cystitis) or kidney infection (pyelonephritis).

So, I was left to ponder:

1. Was my cancer pill causing the problems?

2. Did I have a UTI?

3. Was I pre-diabetic?

4. Had cancer spread to my liver?

5. Were my lymphocytes getting stuck in the lymph nodes?

I'm sure my doctors hated seeing me come. I got a sense they didn't appreciate me doing my own medical research.

You must be your own advocate and research the heck out of everything. Take charge of your own health and ensure your doctors have every piece of information. You might just be saving your own life.

***

Internet Research:

Deciphering Your Lab Report - Testing.com

The U.S. Department of Health and Human Services (HHS) issued a final rule in 2014 that allows patients or their representatives direct access to laboratory test reports after having their identities verified, without the need to have the tests sent to a health practitioner first. This rule is intended to empower you, to allow you to act as a partner with your healthcare provider and take a more active role in your healthcare decisions.

Easier access to test results, however, places you in a position of greater responsibility. You may encounter complex test results on lab reports and will need to recognize that there is a context in which providers use results to make treatment decisions. This may require that you educate yourself about your tests in order to understand their purpose and meaning. Testing.com and other credible sources of health information online can assist you in achieving a better understanding of your medical information.

***

Today's Quote:

"Life wants you to fight it

Learn how to make it your own.

It wants you to grab an axe and hack through the wood.

It wants you to get a sledgehammer and break through concrete.

It wants you to grab a torch and burn through the metal and steel until you can reach through and grab it.

Life wants you to grab all the organized, the alphabetized, the chronological, the sequenced. It wants you to mix it all together,

stir it up,

blend it."

—Colleen Hoover

A Note to You:

My purpose in reviewing my lab results is to encourage you to study your reports. It's easy to feel powerless regarding your health, but reading and understanding lab results can give you the sense that you're in control. Plus, it can be surprisingly fun to research all the weird things written on there! But don't get too scared if you come across something unexpected. Those things that seem like red flags might end up saving your life when you bring them to the attention of your medical team.

Cancer Post #56: How Facebook Nurses Nailed It: July 26th

I shared my lab results on Facebook. I thought they pointed to a urinary tract infection. I immediately had fifteen nurses weighing in with their opinions, and everyone said it looked like a UTI.

I keep preaching about being your own advocate, and I will continue. I left a message at my oncologist's office to please call me back. Later in the afternoon, the nurse called me, asking me what I needed. I began the dialogue by saying, "Please look at the lab report from my ER visit. Many of my Facebook nurse friends think everything points to a UTI."

We went through the lab report line by line, and the nurse noted each abnormal result. After she reviewed the report, I asked, "Do I have a UTI?"

She sighed deeply, "It looks like you do, and also a lung infection. I will discuss this with the doctor and get back to you."

Approximately an hour later, the nurse returned the call, "The doctor can definitively confirm the presence of a lung infection. However, the exact type remains unknown. Fortunately, the medication she prescribed should treat both your UTI and the lung infection."

During my consultation with the nurse, she shared I should expect to undergo significant bodily changes for several months to a year as my body adjusted to the Letrozole medication. The nurse used the analogy of ocean waves to describe the ebbs and flows of these changes.

I concluded the call by asking the nurse to alert my doctor about my dissatisfaction. I was stunned those two infections had slipped past the ER doctor and my oncologist's attention. It wasn't my duty to monitor these things, but apparently, it fell on me. I learned that I should have contacted my general practitioner instead, as these health problems were not related to cancer. I guess the patient should be given a chain of command chart to know who to call when.

I called my daughter Ginger to blow off steam. She advised me to take slow and controlled breaths with my mouth closed, inhaling for four counts before exhaling to the exact count. This technique is meant to expand the lungs and help reduce stress. Ginger even suggested I try propping myself up when lying down so that I could keep the capacity of my lungs inflated. It's incredible how wise advice from those who have been through a situation can teach you what works.

My friend, Margo, a nurse, suggested I take some probiotics to protect me from the backlash caused by the antibiotics. The circle never ends. You fight one illness with another; you only hope the first isn't lurking around, waiting for its chance to strike like an ex-boyfriend in a dark alley.

I fretted that my new husband would be frustrated now that I had more wrong with me, but he remained steadfast and never complained. He proved to be a solid foundation I could count on. I settled down on the couch with a cold glass of cranberry juice and waited to see what tomorrow would bring.

***

Internet Research:

Will you have Urinary tract infection if you take Letrozole? | eHealthMe

We study 47,216 people who have side effects when taking Letrozole. Urinary tract infection is reported by 1,460 (3.09%) of them. People who are more likely to have Urinary tract infection are female, 60+ old, have been taking the drug for 1 - 6 months, also take Kisqali and have High blood pressure.

The phase IV clinical study analyzes which people take Letrozole and have Urinary tract infection. It is created by eHealthMe based on data from the FDA, and is updated regularly.

***

Today's Quote:

"Laughter boosts the immune system and helps the body fight off disease, cancer cells as well as viral, bacterial and other infections. Being happy is the best cure of all diseases!"
—Patch Adams

A Note for You:

Trust your instincts. If you feel your doctor missed something, take the time to look into the results and share them with someone in the medical field. If I had ignored my intuition, I would have continued suffering from an untreated UTI.

Cancer Post #57: Institute of Science: August 3rd

As a COVID Vaccine Test Subject for Moderna, I regularly reported my health to the science institute to help gather data on the vaccine. After filling out my digital health diary and indicating a visit to the emergency room, they promptly scheduled an illness check-up for me.

With each in-car visit to the science institute, my doctor greeted me with an outstretched arm for a warm handshake and the endearing nickname— "Sweetheart."

The team took my blood and vitals, swabbed my nose, and the doctor gave me a physical from the front seat of Neil's car. Talk about curbside service!

The doctor questioned me about the shingles shot. He warned me of the alarming number of individuals who contracted shingles after receiving the COVID-19 vaccine. With a somber tone, he revealed his own wife had been diagnosed with breast cancer at the same time as me. I pressed for information on any potential connection between the vaccine and higher cancer risk; he stated research was underway.

I asked him, "Because I have a lung infection, if I get Covid, what would be the outcome?"

"Sweetheart," he said softly, "Give the medicine time to take effect before you go out into crowds and risk contracting Covid. With a lung infection already present, it could be serious."

Many oppose the vaccine, but I saw it as my duty to participate. My father's bravery during WWII inspired me to contribute meaningfully to the greater good. He had given everything for our nation's liberty, and I wanted to follow in his footsteps. Despite acknowledging the potential dangers, I willingly stepped forward, propelled by my father's values and an unyielding desire to serve my country. This project was a calculated risk that I chose to undertake, prepared for any complications that may arise.

The following day, I debated about returning to work. I awoke at my regular 5 AM time to get ready. However, I thought with my weak immune system and body fighting two infections at once, it probably wasn't a good idea to risk exposing myself to anything nasty while I felt so vulnerable.

When I complained to my husband about yet another setback, he said, "Be careful, you may be sliding into a victim's attitude."

The UTI and lung infection hit me hard emotionally. I repeatedly asked myself whether it was worth it to continue taking that dratted Letrozole pill with all its complications. It stripped away my quality of life. I was consumed by questions and doubts about its benefits versus the side effects.

My friend Darren, the author of With Worn-Out Tools, a memoir about his health issues, asked me what he could do for me. I answered brokenly, "When you see me succumbing to victimhood, please help pull me out from its murky depths."

He said, "Know that we are victors and not victims."

The antibiotic my oncologist put me on was Levofloxacin.

***

Internet Research:

Levofloxacin: Uses, Dosage, Side Effects & Warnings - Drugs.com

Levofloxacin is usually only used for bacterial infections that cannot be treated with safer antibiotics. This is because levofloxacin is a fluoroquinolone (flor-o-KWIN-o-lone) antibiotic and fluoroquinolone antibiotics can cause serious or disabling side effects.

***

Today's Quote:

"Cancer recovery is hard work. Life is hard work. And it really pays off. Hang in there."

—Helen Szablya

A Note to You:

Hey, I know life can be tough, and when it feels like everything is bearing down on you. Just keep walking forward, keep pushing through, and things will get brighter.

Cancer Post: #58: Self-Protection: August 5th

Before cancer, I was never afraid for my health. I worked every day during the Covid shutdown. I ate at restaurants, visited my friends, and never worried about getting the virus.

Cancer created a new normal in my life: fear of cancer returning; and fear of catching a virus. Every time I turned on the news, a reporter mentioned a new strain of COVID-19 to worry about and another booster vaccine to take. Paranoia became my constant companion, lurking in every person who coughed or sneezed near me.

I scrubbed my hands for the fourth time in an hour. The Bible preached against fear, but was it wrong to be cautious? It seemed necessary, keeping me hyper-focused on every surface I touched and everyone approaching within six feet. Perhaps a dose of worry was healthy if it fueled my vigilance in self-protection.

I used to believe those with pre-existing conditions were overly anxious and alarmist about the virus in 2020, but I was wrong. Now I understand the depth of their fear—because I had joined them as one of those vulnerable. Cancer changed my perspective and made me realize how unkind and judgmental my earlier assumptions were. No matter what else this past year has brought, it has taught me an invaluable lesson in compassion.

At one of my appointments with my lymphedema therapist, I mentioned, "Since I had been on antibiotics, my breast didn't feel hard, full, and tender."

My therapist drew a possible connection for me—perhaps the antibiotics had cleared up the inflammation in my breast that had been there all along. I had an ah-ha moment as I realized we must think critically and connect the dots when navigating our healthcare.

***

Internet Research:

COVID-19 and Breast Cancer: What You Need To Know

Since COVID-19 was first identified, the virus has been an added source of stress for many people diagnosed with breast cancer and their loved ones. People with weakened immune systems and certain other conditions are at higher risk for serious illness from COVID-19. But not everyone with a history of breast cancer is at risk for severe COVID, so it's important to talk with your doctors about your individual situation.

***

Today's Quote:

Want to hear a terrible joke? Okay, here we go.

"Did you hear about the bee who had a tumor? Don't worry - it was BEE-nign."

—Anonymous

A Note to You:

It's normal to feel lost with a new symptom. But remember to step back and assess the bigger picture. Are all the pieces of your healthcare puzzle adding up to something others may not see? Don't be afraid to think outside the box; it might lead you to answers.

PEEK-A-BOOB

NOTES AND THOUGHTS

Chapter Eighteen

BREASTIES

Cancer Post #59: Besties in Battle: August 6th

My friend Claudette's doctor called her after her routine mammogram. We both figured it would be a benign fibroid. Further examinations confirmed a diagnosis of breast cancer.

Before we knew of her diagnosis, I already planned on driving to Texas to visit her. I called to ensure she was up for company, and she eagerly expressed joy at my impending arrival. Despite her ability to manage alone, I refused to leave her to grapple with the onslaught of thoughts and questions that come with hearing the words, "You have cancer."

When I arrived at her home, Claudette's face was a picture of serenity. When we sat down for a meal, she cast her eyes downward in prayer, her lips barely moving as she uttered her words of faith. She believed without question that the Lord would save her from whatever ailed her. Claudette did not walk in fear but in peace because of her strong faith. I paled in comparison to Claudette's unwavering devotion and conviction. Still, I remained firm in my own resolve - that God loves me despite my flaws and offerings. Just as many of us have children who are each different, we don't love one more than the other. I feel God would like me to have the same strength of faith as Claudette, but he knows I believe.

We cherished every moment of our time together. Claudette interrogated me, drawing on my experience with cancer. As we nibbled on slivers of cake, we delved into the importance of nutrition. We discussed surgical options and available treatments while also joking about the most comfortable bras. Our conversation flowed between our past, present, and future, filling the room with laughter. Giggling, we donned matching pajamas I brought as a gift to her, and we settled in front of the TV to watch a movie and relax.

Most Doctors don't tell you cancer is as much of a mental challenge as it is physical. The journey ahead can be filled with unknowns and surprises you and your friends may be unprepared for. It is essential to be there for each other. A cancer diagnosis can feel like being lost in a foreign land where you don't understand the language or the signs. Hold each other's hands, literally and figuratively.

When friends offer to assist you, by all means, accept it. Not doing so would deprive your friend of the joy of helping. May you be blessed as both the receiver and the giver. When you help another friend with breast cancer, you become breasties.

***

Internet Research:

What Does That Mean? — Glossary - Rethink Breast Cancer

A "breastie" is a term used in the breast cancer community to describe your breast cancer best friend, combining breast cancer + best friend = breastie!

***

Today's Quote:

"Today will never come again. Be a blessing. Be a friend. Encourage someone. Take time to care. Let your words heal and not wound."

—Unknown

A Note to You:

When your friend is hit with a breast cancer bombshell, don't hesitate to rush to her side. She needs you more than ever; your love and support can make all the difference. As a survivor, I can tell you that having someone who truly understands is crucial on this journey. Let her know she's not alone and that you'll be by her side every step of the way.

PEEK-A-BOOB

NOTES AND THOUGHTS

CHAPTER NINETEEN

FINDING BALANCE IN "JUST FEELING FAIR"

Cancer Post #60: MD Anderson: August 9th

Two months passed since my radiation treatments, yet I still carried the weight of a lead lump. Balancing working full-time and doing basic tasks like running errands felt like insurmountable challenges. My energy and motivation were drained, leaving me feeling nothing but mediocrity.

Every time I got the results of my medical tests, I wondered if the reports were simply filed away without anyone bothering to read them. I felt frustrated and worried about my health. I wanted to ask my oncologist about the follow-up work that needed to be done, but I didn't know which specialist was responsible for what.

With the following battery of upcoming medical tests, I hoped I would get an answer as to why I only felt fair. I hoped something minor and fixable would make me feel good like I did before cancer.

I toyed around with the idea that if the new test results didn't provide me with any answers, I might make an appointment at MD Anderson. I shared my thoughts with a couple of the residents where I work. One of the women who battled cancer claimed she would only go to MD Anderson. With conviction, she said, "They don't play around".

All I knew was my body didn't feel right. My thoughts raced with questions: Was I being irrational? Could a visit to MD Anderson eliminate the fear of constantly wondering if something was wrong, and free me from this anxiety? I wanted to be emancipated from this constant worry about cancer returning so I could focus on living my life.

***

Internet Research:

Why MD Anderson | MD Anderson Cancer Center

We focus exclusively on cancer and have seen cases of every kind. Our doctors treat more rare cancers in a single day than most physicians see in a lifetime. That means you receive expert care no matter your diagnosis.

***

Today's Quote:

"God didn't promise days without pain, laughter without sorrow, or sun without rain, but He did promise strength for the day, comfort for the tears, and light for the way."

—Unknown

A Note to You:

I've spoken to many women who have been to M.D. Anderson. Every one of them has been blown away by their level of care and attention to detail. I suggest looking into it if it brings you some solace. You know how important peace of mind is, especially when everything feels uncertain.

PEEK-A-BOOB

NOTES AND THOUGHTS

CHAPTER TWENTY

GUARDIANS WITHIN: IMMUNE SYSTEM

Cancer Post #61: Goals: August 11th

My recent X-rays revealed two health concerns: an enlarged heart and a lung infection. A nurse at my job confirmed the findings, and I called my oncologist for further testing on both issues. It didn't seem my medical team showed the kind of concern for my problems I thought they should, so I pushed my concerns to the forefront.

The following Monday, I underwent a sonogram to check my heart. I felt greatly relieved when the doctor told me it was completely healthy. Afterward, I called up my friend Luana, who had recently faced her own heart problems. When I shared the good news with her, she exclaimed, "I've known you for years, and you've always had a good heart."

Luana's infectious laughter echoed through the phone, and soon, we were both chuckling.

On Tuesday, I underwent lung X-rays. My intuition told me the worst: lung cancer. Talking became a struggle, every sentence interrupted by violent coughs. My co-worker Kim, who worked in the office beside mine, said, "You sound terrible. You should probably go home."

"Unfortunately, I'm unable to leave at the moment. I promised one of the residents I would help them with a task this afternoon. However, I appreciate your concern and will heed your advice and leave afterward. Thank you for caring," I answered.

I glanced at the clock - 3:30 p.m. I finished and headed out the door to the ER.

The ER doctor tested me for COVID-19, which came back negative. As he was talking to me, I got an email saying the results of my chest X-rays were in. I asked him to check them. He looked it over briefly and said, "You don't have cancer in your lungs," he said.

I let out a huge sigh.

The doctor continued, "It looks like you have had a recent bout of pneumonia. Now you have a respiratory infection."

Interestingly, none of my doctors had mentioned that to me.

"Am I coughing so much because of this respiratory infection," I asked with confusion, "Like an ordinary cold?"

"Well, yes," he said.

"Why do I keep getting sick?"

He explained that my radiation and breast cancer treatments had taken their toll on my immune system. The same thing my boss kept telling me. The ER doctor explained that when I get a cold or infection, it will be more severe than in other people since my immune system doesn't have all guns firing to fight it.

I inquired, "How much longer until my immune system improves? I am sick of being ill, taking time off work, and missing out on life."

He placed his hands on the counter and looked at me solemnly. "It's likely going to take a year, so you should prepare for a bumpy ride as we get closer to winter."

I expressed my gratitude to the doctor and departed for home. I opened the garage door and headed directly to our couch. In minutes, I drifted off to sleep. I turned to sleep as my refuge when defeat consumed me.

I felt like Mrs. Potato Head, with all the plastic parts spread over the floor, broken and jumbled, until I could find the pieces that fit together just right to make me whole again.

I plotted a roadmap to reclaim my life from cancer. My primary objective was to bolster my immunity. Armed with research and insights from YouTube and Dr. Google, I resolved to confront my immune system head-on and achieve victory.

I told my immune system, "Cancer, your evil sure is trying to get the best of me, but we are duking it out, and Cancer, you will lose!"

***

Internet Research:

Here is how I planned to rebuild my immune system. The information is from this website.

How Cancer Patients Can Boost Their Immune System (bensnaturalhealth.com)

1. Eat A Healthy & Nutritious Diet

Focus on a range of healthy foods, including many fruits and vegetables. Many foods and drinks contain germs that may cause infections. Therefore, it is essential to wash raw vegetables and fruits before eating.

I realized I needed to improve my produce-washing habits. Having grown up on a farm, I would casually pick cherries, peaches, apricots, apples, pears, and blackberries straight from the trees in our orchard and eat them. Carrots would come straight out of my dad's garden, with just a quick wipe on my shirt before enjoying their sweet flavor along with the peelings. But now, things are different; I must remember to thoroughly wash all my fruits and vegetables before indulging in them.

2. Sleep Well

An uninterrupted seven hours of sleep per night can make your immune system strong and function well.

3. Observe Proper Hand Hygiene

If you want your immune system to focus on fighting cancer, steer clear of germ-containing places. As cancer treatments weaken your immunity, practicing hand hygiene is essential. Showering and bathing regularly are also necessary.

4. Get Moving

You can help your immune system function well with the positive effects of exercise.

I promised myself I would get some kind of movement at least five days a week. It didn't matter what exercise I chose; my only goal was to do it even if it was dancing to my favorite songs when no one was watching.

5. Report Symptoms of Infection As Soon As Possible

If you suspect any of the following symptoms, you should immediately consult your cancer team:

- Sore throat

- Nasal congestion

- Fever and chills

- Changes in mental status

- Cough

- Diarrhea

- Vomiting

- Swelling or redness in any part of the body.

6. Reduce Stress Levels

Daily stress is very common among cancer patients and is not good for their health. High levels of stress hormones affect the body's ability to defend itself and suppress immune function.

7. Avoid Unhealthy Foods and Drinks

There's no doubt that unhealthy and refined foods can weaken your immune system. Unhealthy fats, refined sugars, processed and charred meats, and alcohol intake are highly restricted for cancer patients undergoing immunotherapy and other treatments.

8. Avoid Contact with People Who Have an Infection

Cancer patients must avoid spending time with people who have flu, fever, or other infections.

***

Today's Quote:

"People with a strong willpower will always have the bigger picture in mind. They will be able to forgo small pleasures in order to help attain bigger goals."

—Bryan Adams

A Note to You:

The power to create your own path lies within you. You are the master of your destiny, and no one can take that from you. These trials may seem daunting, but you will succeed.

PEEK-A-BOOB

NOTES AND THOUGHTS

Chapter Twenty-One

OVERCOMING THE STRUGGLE OF SELF

Cancer Post #62: Mirror of Misgivings: August 12th

Cancer left me embarrassed of my body. The scars on my breast were bearable, but it was the swelling in my abdomen brought on by Letrozole that I could not get used to. All my pretty clothes mocked me, as every item seemed to crease and strain around my belly rolls. Even when I managed to squeeze myself into a dress, I couldn't stand the sight of myself in the mirror afterward. My changed body thrust me into an unfamiliar world of body shaming.

My advanced years, cancer and Letrozole combined, aged me rapidly. How could I be good to my body with all the hate I felt?

I realized I needed to love myself. Hate wouldn't motivate me, but love would drive me. I committed to treating my body with respect. To feel attractive and confident, I couldn't overlook the importance of wearing clothes that fit well in a larger size. Instead of trying to hate my body into shape, I had to approach this journey with affection and care.

I had a clear vision of my purpose, my WHY. I knew I wanted to leave a legacy of resilience and determination for my children and grandchildren. Losing weight was essential in preventing cancer recurrence. I wanted Neil to be proud to be seen with me and set an example for my grown children, two bonus daughters, and grandchildren. That was my driving force, my WHY.

I scrutinized my reflection in the bathroom mirror, taking note of my thick waist, flabby arms, and stubborn extra pounds. A fierce determination ignited within me to make a drastic change for my health goals. I made a conscious decision to love and embrace myself wholly and unconditionally. I committed myself to an internal transformation.

After hours of researching different weight-loss techniques, I finally put together my own plan. I knew it would work if I remained consistent.

- I started with a 1400-calorie-a-day diet.
- I ate more vegetables and fruits and less meat, pasta, dairy, and sweets.
- I allowed for one cheat day a month.
- I drank eight glasses of water daily.

I want to share the correlation between Letrozole and weight gain for today's research.

***

Internet Research:

Does Letrozole Cause Weight Gain? (survivingbreastcancer.org)

One factor that is seldom discussed (and more research is certainly warranted) is the role that Letrozole has on lipid metabolism. While there have been some trials and research investigating the impact aromatase inhibitors have on the lipid profile, results have been elusive [5]. What we do understand is that these AI's can have an adverse effect on blood levels. For example, increasing total cholesterol, LDL (the "bad" cholesterol) and HDL (the "good" cholesterol) levels can lead to increased risk of cardiovascular disease [6]. Additionally, we know that the enzyme lipoprotein lipase (LPL), which is controlled by insulin, pulls fat out of the bloodstream and into the cell. If this enzyme is on a muscle cell, it will turn the fat into energy. If the enzyme is sitting on a fat cell, it will pull fat into the cell and make it fatter [7]. Estrogen suppresses LDL and with lower levels of estrogen in the body, this could be a reason some women gain weight during menopause or as part of breast cancer treatment.

***

Today's Quote or a Bit of Sarcasm:

"The patient's medical history has been remarkably insignificant, with only a 40-pound weight gain in the last three days."

—Unknown

My Note to You:

We cannot truly excel unless we first love ourselves wholly and unconditionally. Embrace every part of yourself, even the bits that may seem imperfect. Turn those self-criticisms into affirmations of self-love. When setting goals, remember to connect with your inner why. Sending love and light to all my pink sisters.

Cancer Post #63: Embracing the Sweat: August 13th

Neil and I had always talked about traveling and seeing the world. He wanted to take me to beautiful European cities, explore every inch of Nashville, and walk on the beach at sunset in Destin, Florida. I knew I had to get back in shape to do those things. The choice to exercise or not was mine. If I didn't exert myself regularly, my body would wither away like a flower, and I would never be strong. The kind of future my new husband and I had depended on my choices today, not yesterday or tomorrow.

My plan for a strong body:
- Walk five days a week.
- YouTube stretches for senior citizens five mornings a week.
- Join the Livestrong program at the YMCA.
- I allow for one lazy day a month. I could just veg out and watch Netflix if that is what I wanted to do.

The recent X-rays I had showed degenerative changes in my thoracic spine and shoulders. Degenerative changes in the spine mean that there is some loss of bone in the spine. Degenerative shoulder problems are caused by wear and tear of the soft tissue in the shoulder. Exercise will help these degenerative changes.

***

Internet Research:

Four Things You Should Know about LIVESTRONG at the YMCA | by Livestrong | Livestrong Voices

The LIVESTRONG at the YMCA program is a 12-week, evidence-based physical activity program designed with the goal of getting cancer survivors back on their feet. Facilitated by specially certified instructors, the program includes two 75–90-minute sessions per week, which implement a combination of cardiovascular conditioning, strength training, balance, and flexibility exercise. Instructors are trained in cancer survivorship, post-rehabilitation exercise and supportive cancer care. It is open to adults 18 years or older, and is currently offered for free at more than 650 YMCA branches across 41 states in the US.

***

Today's Quote: Top Ten Ways to Know You Are a Cancer Thriver

1 "Your alarm clock goes off at 6 a.m., and you're glad to hear it."

2. "Your mother-in-law invites you to lunch, and you say NO."

3. "You're back in the family rotation to take out the garbage."

4. "When you no longer have an urge to choke the person who says, "all you need to beat cancer is the right attitude."

5. "When your dental floss runs out, and you buy 1000 yards."

6. "When you use your toothbrush to brush your teeth and not comb your hair."

7. "You have a chance to buy additional life insurance, but you buy a new convertible car instead."

8. "Your doctor tells you to lose weight and do something about your cholesterol, and you listen."

9. "When your biggest annual celebration is again your birthday and not the day you were diagnosed."

10. "When you use your Visa card more than your hospital parking pass."

—Anonymous

A Note for You:

C'mon, let's do this. I know you hate hearing it, and I feel the same way, but we both know how good we'll feel after! Let's just make the most of it and become one of those people who actually enjoy exercising.

Cancer Post #64: Reclaiming My Dreams: August 15th

I took back what cancer took away. It felt powerful to regain my immune system, lose weight, get into an exercise routine, and set goals. But most importantly for me, I wanted to pursue my biggest dream once again. I challenge you to identify four things that have been lost over your life's journey. It doesn't matter if it is from cancer, another illness, depression, or procrastination. Your next step is to plan how to recover what got lost along the way. Then put it all into action—watch out, world!

My dream is to become a writer whose words make an impact. At age twelve, I pried open a book on a cold December afternoon. I read a scene where a grandfather gave a butterscotch candy to his grandson. The author's precise and impassioned description of the simple confection made my mouth water. I felt the butterscotch flavor on my tongue. With that book open on my lap and the desire for a piece of candy wrapped in gold foil, I realized the immense power of words.

Filled with a burning desire, I transformed my Facebook posts about my battle with cancer into a book that could shed light on the unspoken truths. This dream gave me renewed energy and purpose.

Let's take back our dreams!

***

Internet Research:

Goal setting during your cancer journey (piedmont.org)

Goal setting can keep you motivated, focused, and empowered during your cancer journey.

"Goal setting helps us be present and move forward," says Lauren Garvey, MS, CRC, NCC, a counselor and facilitator at Cancer Wellness at Piedmont. "A forward mindset and positivity are very important, especially during cancer treatment."

***

Today's Quote:

"If you set goals and go after them with all the determination you can muster, your gifts will take you places that will amaze you."

—Les Brown

A Note to You:

My dear friend, I know how difficult it must be to battle cancer, but don't lose sight of your future. Take a moment to envision your goals and write them down. It takes courage, but it will bring you hope and determination. Believe in yourself; anything you set your heart and mind to, you can accomplish. Don't let any obstacles stop you. Find your inner drive and make an action plan. Don't make excuses. As you set your goals, be patient with yourself and celebrate every effort you make towards reaching them. Don't expect perfection; just keep moving forward. Remember to prioritize self-care as a goal. Be grateful for the strength that allows you to work towards your aspirations. And finally, celebrate each milestone along the way by breaking your objectives into smaller, achievable steps. You can do it!

Cancer Post #65: The Bliss of Feeling Good: August 19th

While walking from the employee parking lot to my work building a gentle breeze stirred, and a shaft of sunlight warmed my shoulder as someone approached me. The lady looked me in the eyes and asked how I was feeling. My lips curved up into a genuine grin. My soul felt light for the first time since June 1st, and I replied "Good" with conviction. The world around me sparkled just a little bit more brightly.

    A renewed energy returned to me, and I felt normal for the first time in months. The oppressive nausea from the Letrozole had dissipated on this day, leaving me with a newfound appreciation for feeling well. I vowed never to take this feeling of health for granted again, for it could disappear as quickly as it had arrived.

    Setting achievable goals proved to be the key to improving my well-being. After one week of diligently following my plans, I noticed a significant change - I had shed two pounds! I kept hydrated by drinking eight glasses of water daily and pushed myself to meet my exercise targets. Prioritizing my dreams and actively pursuing them became a daily habit for me.

    I celebrated an entire week without catching some infection that would make me miss work. My new habits could be key in returning me to the Shelley I was before breast cancer.

***

Internet Research:

How Surgery Affects the Immune System (breastcancer.org)

Breast cancer surgery also can challenge your immune system for a couple of other reasons: Surgery breaks the skin and underlying tissues, which can allow bacteria and germs to enter the body. If an infection happens, it can occur right away or during the healing process. Once the incision heals, the risk of local infection goes away. During surgery to treat the cancer, your doctor usually removes a few or more of the underarm lymph nodes so they can be checked for the presence of breast cancer cells. If cancer cells are found, more lymph nodes may need to be removed. (For more information, see the Lymph Node Removal section. Lymph nodes play a key role in filtering out bacteria and other harmful substances while also exposing them to infection-fighting white blood cells and triggering an immune response. The more lymph nodes you have removed, the greater the disruption to your immune system. Any cut, bug bite, burn, or other injury that breaks the skin on the arm, hand, or trunk on that side of your body can challenge the immune system and possibly lead to infection. This risk never really goes away.

***

Today's Quote:

"The mind, in addition to medicine, has powers to turn the immune system around."

—Jonas Salk

My Note to You:

My dear pink sister, hold onto hope. One day soon, you will feel the light within you shine once more. And when it does, dance under the stars and celebrate your journey of self-discovery and growth.

Cancer Post #66: Mindset Mastery: August 21st

I gained insight into mindset in an online seminar with my P31 network. The guest lecturer was a physician, board-accredited in medical oncology and internal medication.

He discussed many critical points about cancer. However, one of his comments caused me to spend the next few days soaking it in and taking it to heart. He said, "Cancer is your enemy. Whatever treatment you are taking to stop cancer is your friend."

He described the purpose of aromatase inhibitors. The doctor reminded us mindset was vital in surviving cancer. I complained a lot about the side effects Letrozole caused me in previous chapters. This doctor helped me understand I needed to remember cancer was the enemy, and my tiny yellow pill was my friend, working hard to keep a recurrence at bay. The doctor also suggested, "Don't fight the drug that fights cancer."

The doctor's words were sobering yet also filled with a glimmer of hope. He told us cancer cells were so small it would take one billion to be visible on a mammogram. He mentioned studies showing that women taking aromatase inhibitors had fewer chances of recurrence. But then his voice dropped as he warned us that these tiny cells could get into the blood and cause damage.

The doctor finished his Zoom call with determination in his voice. He reiterated that even when we can't seem to find the strength to eat right, exercise, rest, and reduce stress, that is where our willpower comes into play. His words were laden with compassion as he said, "You need physical and emotional healing from cancer."

***

Internet Research:

Can altering cancer 'mindsets' change physical outcomes? - Scope (stanford.edu)

They theorized that adopting a mindset change about cancer from "cancer is a catastrophe" to "cancer is manageable," or about the body ('My body is capable' vs 'my body is an adversary') could be transformative.

***

Today's Quote:

"Believe you can, and you are halfway there."

—Theodore Roosevelt

A Note to You:

When the weight of the world feels like it's crushing you, and even the simplest tasks seem insurmountable, try to do something-anything-just for yourself. It could be sipping a soothing herbal tea, or spending a few minutes of doing gentle stretching. Sometimes, you only need a hug and a little shift in your mindset to make everything more manageable. Hugs to you, my sweet friend, from me.

NOTES AND THOUGHTS

Chapter Twenty-Two

LADY PARTS AND WEIGHT GAIN

Cancer Post #67: Sacred Spaces: August 22nd

At the age of sixty-five, my physician informed me that I no longer required a pap smear. Because of the breast cancer, I worried there could be cancer elsewhere in my body. I asked my primary care doctor for an appointment to have a pap smear. I wasn't looking for any more tumors. I just wanted comfort in knowing my down south lady parts were healthy. Upon my primary care doctor's referral, I booked an appointment with a gynecologist.

A sweet receptionist greeted me upon my arrival. The waiting room felt calm and serene, with soft pink hues against white walls. Cozy furniture complemented the ambiance.

I was given a soft, fuzzy robe to put on. The robe smelled like fresh air, honey, and warm sunshine. It was a cheerful yellow color with designs in the print. I told the doctor that having such a pretty wrap made me feel cared for. She explained her mother told her those paper gowns you get in the doctor's offices make you feel yucky just putting them on. Her mother made dozens of robes so her patients could experience a pampered feeling. This kindness made me feel valued as a person. I told her I was obsessed with ensuring all cancer was gone everywhere. I stated, "I know Medicare no longer thinks I need pap smears, but please don't treat me for my age, but treat me for the person I am and my needs."

I added, "Doctor, my best friend's sister-in-law was eighty when she died from ovarian cancer, and if Medicare thinks people of that age are too old to get it, they are wrong. I need to know for my peace of mind that my uterus and ovaries are cancer-free."

The doctor must have seen the anxiety on my face and asked, "Do you want us to do an ultrasound? That way, we can check for ovarian or cervical cancer. It might make you feel more secure if we do it, but I don't want to pressure you into something that might be too much. What do you think?"

"Yes," I confirmed, "When I know my lady parts are healthy, I will be reassured of my odds for survival. Thank you."

She scheduled an ultrasound for September. Checking all my parts out brought me tranquility. Each person is different in their needs on this journey. I have a detail-oriented, sometimes pain-in-the-butt personality. I had to know all the bases were covered and an action plan was in place.

***

Internet Research:

(How often should a woman over 65 have a Pap smear? | UnitedHealthcare (uhc.com)

As many as 20% of cervical cancer cases occur in women aged 65 and older, according to research out of the University of Alabama at Birmingham. Study results also showed that the rate of cervical cancer diagnosis was higher in women age 70 – 79 than in women age 20 – 29. Prior to these findings, the view was that cervical cancer was usually only diagnosed in younger women. The outlook for cervical cancer is favorable when the disease is caught early, and regular Pap smear tests are the key to early diagnosis.

***

Today's Quote:

"It's about focusing on the fight and not the fright."

—Robin Roberts

A Note to You:

Dear Pink Sisters, I understand the crippling fear of wondering if your cancer has spread beyond what you already know. But you are strong and brave enough to talk to your doctors about it. Don't let them brush away your fears - if you feel like cancer cells are lurking elsewhere, tell your medical team you want something done about it. You have been through so much already; worrying constantly about other cancer cells is a life no one deserves. Take control of your body, stand up for yourself, and don't give up until they listen.

Cancer Post #68: Battling the Bulge: August 23rd

Calories Consumed: 1,205
　Fit Bit Calories Out: 1,932
　Steps: 12,650
　Today's Healthy Eating Tip:
Brain cells come and brain cells go, but fat cells live forever.

　My heart sank with disappointment. I diligently adhered to my diet for twelve days, but the scale showed no change. Determined to understand how this cancer pill affected my weight, I needed to pinpoint the necessary adjustments to shed some pounds. Frustration made me want to give up, but I wouldn't allow frustration to win.

***

Internet Research:

Weight Gain | Cancer.Net

Hormonal therapy may be used to treat certain cancers, including breast, prostate, testicular, and uterine cancers. This type of medication can decrease the amount of certain hormones, such as estrogen, progesterone, or testosterone. Hormones in the body are used for different functions. Decreases in hormone levels can increase fat, decrease muscle, and make it harder to burn calories.

***

Today's Quote from Howard:

My friend Howard from New York knew I was about to give up, so he texted me this perfect quote to keep me motivated.

"If I quit now, I will be back to where I started, and when I started, I was desperately wishing to be where I am now."

—Anonymous

A Note to You:

My dear friend, if you're struggling with weight gain, I understand the emotional pain it causes us. While people tell us, "At least you're alive, a few pounds won't matter."

Our well-meaning friends don't fully comprehend the situation. The fat creates more estrogen, something we must avoid to prevent recurrence. It's so hard when friends bring us tempting treats! Let's thank them and give the high-calorie gifts to our neighbors or even throw the sweets in the trash can instead of succumbing to temptation. On top of everything else, extra weight can lead to depression. Hang in there! Veggies and fruits are our allies in this fight, and sweets are nothing more than temporary enemies. It's best not to be around the sweet stuff while taking these meds!

Cancer Post #69: Work That Body: August 30th

I walked into the bright and clean Mitch Park YMCA, my sneakers squeaking on the freshly polished tile floors. My heart thumped with anticipation of my debut in the Livestrong class. With each step closer to the room where others were already congregating, I breathed deeply, feeling a sense of hope that soon, I'd be able to again build muscle strength.

As a breast cancer survivor, I could bring someone to support me. Luckily, my husband Neil joined me. We mingled with the other participants for an icebreaker game, which helped ease the initial tension. By the end of the first class, all of us were giving and getting support from each other. A playful energy permeated the atmosphere.

The women surrounding me astounded me with their vibrant energy and unbreakable determination. But one woman in particular stood out to me - Sally. Despite her recent chemo treatments, she exuded a powerful aura of strength and confidence. Her recently bald head now sported a chic short style, framing her face and accentuating her regal posture. She greeted each newcomer with open arms, and her unwavering smile lit up the room.

A sense of gratitude filled me at the prospect of this twelve-week free fitness program offered by the YMCA. I could barely contain my excitement as I imagined the potential of transformation and strength this incredible gift would bring to my body.

For the second class, we underwent the grueling process of establishing our physical baseline and pushing ourselves beyond our limits. This baseline would serve as a benchmark of our progress over the next twelve weeks, a testament to the undeniable strength and willpower we gained at the end of the program.

***

Internet Research:

Physical Activity and Cancer Fact Sheet - NCI

Breast cancer: Many studies have shown that physically active women have a lower risk of breast cancer than inactive women. In a 2016 meta-analysis that included 38 cohort studies, the most physically active women had a 12–21% lower risk of breast cancer than those who were least physically active. Physical activity has been associated with similar reductions in risk of breast cancer among both premenopausal and postmenopausal women. Women who increase their physical activity after menopause may also have a lower risk of breast cancer than women who do not.

***

Today's Quote:

"You didn't make it through surgery, radiation, and / or chemo just to end up on the couch. Get an exercise program and get moving!"

—Unknown

A Note to You:

Hey friend, I wanted to remind you of something our Livestrong coach said. Do NOT skip those days when you don't feel like exercising! I know it can be challenging, but on the days that I was feeling unmotivated but dragged myself out to exercise anyway, I felt so much better after the workout. Remember that when you don't want to go - it'll make all the difference if you do go.

PEEK-A-BOOB

NOTES AND THOUGHTS

Chapter Twenty-Three
TRIALS AND DECISIONS

Cancer Post #70: Clinical Trials: August 28th

I have a friend who has Leukemia. She is part of a clinical trial. As we talked, we both thought it valuable to tell her story. She has asked not to be named, but she is generous in sharing her journey.

The study is testing the addition of a new anti-cancer drug, Venetoclax, to the usual treatment (Ibrutinib and Obinutuzumab) in untreated, older patients with Chronic Lymphocytic Leukemia.

The study she is in has public funding from the National Cancer Institute. She can change her mind at any time. The study is being done to answer the following questions:

1. Is adding a new anti-cancer drug to the usual treatment better, the same as, or worse than the usual treatment alone for untreated older patients?

2. Can patients who have no detectable CLL, after a year of receiving the usual treatment plus the new anti-cancer drug, discontinue therapy?

This study has two main study groups. A computer randomly decides the participant's placement in either group one or two. Her research group is for fifteen, 28-day cycles. The infusions, the Obinutuzumab, are given to her for six, twenty-eight-day cycles. She has completed three cycles. She will finish the infusions in November. Once the infusions conclude, she will continue taking the three Ibrutinib chemo pills until next August or September. Possibly for the rest of her life.

In the first 28-day cycle in June, she received four infusions of Obinutuzumab and two or three Hydration infusions. For July & August, she received only one infusion of Obinutuzumab.

The next three will also be only one infusion. She will take the Ibrutinib (3 pills) every day and keep a log of when she takes them. She will give the log to the nurse at the end of each cycle, and the nurse will then give her medications for the following sequence. She will return the extra pills in their original bottle.

After she finishes this study treatment, her doctor will continue to monitor her condition for ten years to watch for side effects and see if her disease worsens. She will visit her doctor every three months for six years and every six months for the remaining four years.

The risks my friend is taking by being in the study are:

1. The drug may not be as good as the usual approach.
2. She could have side effects.

The most common side effects the study doctors know about are:

1. Bruising, joint pain, diarrhea, heartburn, and rash.
2. Atrial fibrillation.
3. Fever, chills, shortness of breath, nausea, chest pain, or low blood pressure.
4. Tumor lysis syndrome, where the cancer cells break down quickly and can release toxins into the bloodstream.
5. Lowering of the neutrophil count, which can lead to infection.

All these therapies are already approved by the FDA for use in chronic lymphocytic leukemia.

There were about 418 people taking part in this study.

Thank you, my friend, for being a hero who will lead to progress in cancer treatments.

At this writing, my friend is in the usual approach but will find out if adding Venetoclax is a better way to go. She has no reported side effects.

***

Internet Research:

Why you should ask about cancer clinical trials - Mayo Clinic Comprehensive Cancer Center Blog

Clinical trials, also known as clinical studies, help medical researchers understand how to diagnose, treat and prevent cancer and other diseases and conditions. Their findings often translate to treatments that can lead to longer, healthier lives for people with cancer.

"Treatment for breast cancer has improved significantly in the past few decades, and these improvements came from clinical trials," says Saranya Chumsri, M.D., a medical oncologist with the Robert and Monica Jacoby Center for Breast Health at Mayo Clinic. "Clinical trials are an important way to learn about new treatments."

***

Today's Quote:

"I think a hero is any person really intent on making this a better place for all people."

—Maya Angelou

A Note to You:

I volunteered to participate in a clinical trial for the Moderna vaccine against COVID-19, and it was an incredible experience. I'm filled with admiration and gratitude for anyone who takes on this challenge, so if you ever decide to join a clinical trial, please know that I'm right alongside you, applauding your courage and tenacity. Thank you for doing your part to help us find better treatments or even a cure!

NOTES AND THOUGHTS

Chapter Twenty-Four

CANCER WINS WHEN

Cancer Post #71: Understanding When Cancer Wins: September 6th

I had a lengthy list of questions ready during my most recent oncology appointment. One was about what kind of food I should be eating, and my oncologist's answer gave me pause and made me think deeply about my choices.

I asked her, "How can I attain a balance between eating only foods that benefit my body and occasionally eating foods I really love?" She paused and looked at me. Her eyes were on fire with passion. "Cancer wins when you don't live your life!"

A moment of realization washed over me, and I finally comprehended. Moving forward, I prioritized making healthier choices most of the time, but did not completely depriving myself. It was okay to indulge in a slice of cake and wine on special occasions; I deserved it.

The oncologist presented the research to me, which said that losing weight could help reduce the risk of breast cancer. She suggested I try to lose between ten and twenty pounds, but warned me it would be difficult due to my medication.

The lab results on my CBC filled me with mixed emotions. The white blood cell count was within normal range, but the red blood cell count was low and signaled anemia. I started taking iron supplements daily, and in a few months, I would have the levels rechecked.

I told my oncologist about my declining memory and how worried I was that this would eventually lead to dementia, just like it did with so many of my family members before me. The doctor reassured me that the changes were due to the Letrozole. My doctor told me my memory would probably improve over time as my body adjusted to its blocking of estrogen. Even so, the fear that I may be next in my family line to inherit memory loss haunted me.

I revealed to my doctor the large number of vitamins I had self-prescribed and consumed. She shook her head, convinced that a healthy diet was all the nourishment I needed and that any supplements were a waste of money. But something in my gut told me the vitamins worked, and no matter what she said, I continued taking them.

A common side effect of taking aromatase inhibitors is a decrease in sexual desire. As a newlywed, this change in my libido required honest and intimate conversations with my husband. This topic will be examined in more detail later on in the book.

The final question I asked my oncologist was, "What do you predict for my life span?"

She spoke, "I can only speculate for the next five years. If you take your Letrozole as prescribed, stay active and lose excess weight, eat right mostly, have some downtime, and limit stress, I can safely say I don't believe you will have a recurrence in the next five years."

With a grin, she added, "Do all of these things, and you should expect to live a regular life expectancy."

I told my friends, "When I refuse the dessert you made or walk away from drama, take a nap, or go to the YMCA instead of the happy hour you invited me to, please know it has nothing to do with you. These are the habits that will keep me strong in the face of my cancer. I am doing these things so I can live a normal life span and beat cancer out of taking me to an early grave."

***

Internet Research:

10 Tips on How to Survive Cancer (verywellhealth.com)

This point may seem obvious to many, but it's important to cover. Seeing an oncologist (a healthcare provider who specializes in diagnosing and treating cancer) is the best way to get the right treatment for your cancer.

***

Today's Quote:

"Cancer is not a death sentence, but rather it is a life sentence; it pushes one to live."

—Marcia Smith

A Note to You:

My oncologist taught me that cancer can win by stealing all the joy in our lives. That's why I think it's important that we take the time to relish those moments without guilt! We shouldn't let cancer take away something that brings us happiness, even if it means going against what we were told to do. It took me a while to understand this, but now I realize that cancer hasn't won when I allow myself to savor life's little pleasures.

NOTES AND THOUGHTS

Chapter Twenty-Five

DOWN THERE

Cancer Post #72: A Continuation: September 7th

Disbelief and shock hit me right in the gut.

I sat anxiously in the hospital exam room, waiting for my ovaries and uterine sonogram. I repeatedly assured myself the tests would reveal nothing, but fear still seeped through my veins like poison. I followed the instructions to a tee, drinking forty-eight ounces of water and fighting off every urge to empty my bladder. The technician warmed up the jelly with practiced ease. As the wand slowly moved across my body, it felt like an eternity until, finally, she said, "You have some gas making your ovaries hard to find. Would you be okay with me doing a transvaginal ultrasound?"

She showed me an instrument that resembled an elongated vibrator. She explained she'd need to insert it inside me for better visuals. All I could think was, how would I keep from urinating all over this exam table with such a full bladder? I guess she read my thoughts. She said, "You can go to the bathroom before we begin."

I rushed to the restroom just in time. I felt like an actress in one of those gotta go commercials.

When I climbed back on the exam table, I looked at the instrument and asked, "Would you mind going slow when you put that inside of me? My vagina is pretty dry right now due to a pill I am taking called Letrozole."

Her face went blank when I mentioned Letrozole. As I explained the cancer pill to her, my frustration built. Why wasn't this common knowledge among the lab technicians who were dealing with breast cancer patients every day?

As the technician inserted the wand, I felt a mixture of relief and apprehension. This test was taking longer than expected, and I desperately wanted to hear that it was all normal. Thank goodness, the test was not painful or uncomfortable. I asked the technician if she could tell me anything while she worked. She said the radiologist would read it, and the report would be on my portal by evening.

When I returned home, I put on my gym clothes and headed to Livestrong class. Neil didn't go with me to the Thursday night classes. Neil got together with his buddy Bill on Thursdays. I felt he needed time away from cancer talk, to drink a beer, and talk sports.

My phone dinged as I was ready to leave for the YMCA. I could access the report on my portal now.

A 1.9 x 1.1 0.0 cm echogenic soft tissue focus in the right adnexal region could represent a mass arising from the right ovary or the adjacent uterus. If clinically indicated, CT with IV contrast material would be helpful for further evaluation.

After reading the test results, I couldn't hold back my tears. Once I reached the YMCA, I immediately shared the news with my Livestrong group. They showed me so much care and kindness, offering hugs and words of encouragement. Despite my body's attempts to weaken me, I remained determined to maintain my health and strength.

I decided not to tell my children or wasband, Horace, of the results. Horace fractured his hip and was experiencing tremendous pain. His surgery was in four days. I needed to be able to help.

I planned to share the news with my kids and Horace when he recovered from his hip operation. I confided in my sister, given that she was familiar with all of the bumps and emotional ups and downs associated with cancer.

When I returned from the YMCA, Neil was already home. I told him what the radiology report showed. His strong arms wrapped around me. He looked into my eyes and vowed that if the news was good, we would celebrate and whoop it up. If it wasn't, we would face it together and kick cancer's butt again.

My primary care doctor called me the following day and said the mass appeared harmless. She reminded me a few weeks prior; no cancer markers were present in my blood tests. On September 21st, I would have a biopsy to verify no cancer cells were in the mass. I promised myself I would not give into despair. I would embrace hope for a positive outcome.

***

Internet Research:

Transvaginal Ultrasound: Purpose, Procedure, and Results (healthline.com)

An ultrasound test uses high-frequency sound waves to create images of your internal organs. Imaging tests can identify abnormalities and help doctors diagnose conditions. A transvaginal ultrasound, also called an endovaginal ultrasound, is a type of pelvic ultrasound used by doctors to examine female reproductive organs. This includes the uterus, fallopian tubes, ovaries, cervix, and vagina. "Transvaginal" means "through the vagina." This is an internal examination.

***

Today's Quote:

"I had uterine cancer, which is the most under-funded and under-researched of all the female cancer."

—Fran Drescher

A Note to You:

It's totally normal to be worried about cancer spreading. Take care of yourself, and don't hesitate to ask for more tests if you feel uneasy. We both know how stress can mess with our bodies, so make a list of things giving you grief and find a way to kick them to the curb. I'm sending you lots of love and hugs.

Cancer Post #73: Smart Alec: September 9th

The office manager at my gynecologist's office called and said the doctor wanted me to get a blood draw at the clinic that day. I informed my boss I would be absent for some time due to additional tests. Unfortunately, the technician struggled to find a suitable vein. Just the day before, blood samples were taken at the science institute as part of my two-year commitment to vaccine research. As the tech drew my blood at the clinic, she raised one eyebrow in surprise and asked, "Have you had a recent experience with needles in your veins?"

I was tempted to be a smart aleck and reply, "Oh yes, I took my daily dose of heroin yesterday."

I resisted the urge to joke around and kept quiet. I knew this visit would become part of my medical record. I told the tech what had caused the raised red bump on my arm. She fumbled with her equipment. On her first try, the tube to hold the blood broke. On her second attempt, my vein rolled away from the needle. Her third try was a charm.

My blood underwent enzyme testing as a part of detecting any uterine cancer. Urine and blood tests were conducted to evaluate the presence of abnormalities in cell structures, hormones, and other substances present that could generate signs of malignancy. The procedure is also utilized to exclude any other possible medical complications.

My doctor explained when the results came back, she would check them for enzymes that may point to uterine cancer. She would follow up with a biopsy.

The doctor reassured me by adding, "The mass is small, only about an inch big. In my years of practice, most of those turn out to be benign."

Again, the waiting game started.

***

Internet Research:

12 Powerful Uterine Cancer Symptoms (veryhealthy.life)

Uterine cancer is one of the five most common cancers that women are diagnosed with, and it's one of the cancers that carry the harshest prognosis. If you suspect that you might be suffering from uterine cancer, your first step is to take a closer look and document your symptoms as they happen. For some, it helps to keep a notebook of their symptoms over time – this is useful for their doctor when diagnosing what could be wrong. Your next step is to take your combined list of symptoms and visit a doctor:

***

Today's Quote:

"You are not defined by your test results. You are so much more than that."

—Unknown

A Note to You:

A word of caution. When you're feeling sassy, like I was when the technician questioned about my veins, it's better to stay silent. Most of the stuff that comes out of your mouth, even if it was meant as a joke, will end up in your medical records.

Cancer Post #74: Three-Month Cancer-Free Party: September 10th

It was a moment of pure happiness as I celebrated my three-month cancer-free milestone surrounded by my loving husband and our close-knit wine club friends. Mary and Roger, who hosted the group, prepared a special place of honor for Neil and me to sit. With her infectious smile, Mary came to where we were sitting and stood in front of us. Proudly, she announced, "Neil and Shelley, the wine club has purchased a special French Champagne in honor of your marriage and your three-month cancer-free celebration."

I watched the champagne being slowly poured into each glass, the sweet fragance filling the air. Our friends clinked their glasses together in a toast, and I smiled, feeling the warmth of friendship and love flooding my heart and knowing this moment would stay with me forever.

Neil and I distributed the most recent edition of CAREGIVER magazine. We surprised our wine club friends by showing a photo of their beaming faces. The magazine published an article about our groovy senior citizen wedding and picked a photo of our zany group to publish.

We pulled out a box of bright pink bracelets we had brought and offered them to the wine club members. The powerful cancer ribbon was conspicuously emblazoned on each bracelet, interwoven with calligraphy that declared hope, strength, faith, and courage in a beautiful display against the vibrant pink rubber. My heart swelled with pride as I watched all of them slip the bracelet on their wrists.

As the night came to a close, we cheered and smiled as we sliced into the pink cake, poured more glasses of wine, and chuckled until our stomachs hurt.

Internet Research:

History of the Pink Ribbon - Breast Cancer Action (bcaction.org)

From the beginning, the pink ribbon connoting breast cancer awareness has been embroiled in controversy. Today, some members of the movement wear it proudly, giving thanks for both the symbol and its attendant charity-dollar largesse. Others hate it with a passion. But to much of the media and the world at large, the ribbon is the breast cancer movement. Where did the ribbon come from, where is it going, and what has it meant along the way?

First on the scene was the Susan G. Komen Breast Cancer Foundation. Komen had been handing out bright pink visors to breast cancer survivors running in its Race for the Cure since late 1990. In fall 1991, mere months after Irons' electrifying appearance, the foundation gave out pink ribbons to every participant in its New York City race.

This first use of the ribbon, though, was for Komen just a detail in the larger and more important story of the race. To really break out, the pink ribbon would need a situation in which the ribbon was the event.
And it didn't take long for that situation to arrive. Early in 1992, Alexandra Penney, then the editor in chief of Self, was busy designing the magazine's second annual Breast Cancer Awareness Month issue. The previous year's effort, inspired and guest edited by Evelyn Lauder—Estée Lauder senior corporate vice president and a breast cancer survivor—had been a huge hit. The question was, how to do it again and even better. Then Penney had a flash of inspiration—she would create a ribbon, and enlist the cosmetics giant to distribute it in New York City stores. Evelyn Lauder went her one better: She promised to put the ribbon on cosmetics counters across the country.

***

Today's Quote:

"It is not so much our friends' help that helps us as the confident knowledge that they will help us."

—Epicurus

A Note for You:

Once we battle the beast that is cancer, our friends and relationships take on a new, profound meaning. Know this: some of your friends will be solid rocks for you to lean on, while other people in your life might unexpectedly retreat. With this knowledge comes clarity; you'll know who your true friends are. When you recognize that select group of people, hold them close and cherish their strength.

Cancer Post #75: Staring Cancer in The Faith: September 12th

A new class started at a local church titled "Staring Cancer in the Faith." Jane Wilson and Sarah McLean wrote the study guide. Their book is available on Amazon. The class focused on the emotional and spiritual healing of breast cancer survivors. I needed this class. I had a lot of back and forth with God on the subject of cancer. I had been tested. My faith had been tested.

Some of the topics explored were:
- I'm Still Here, But I'm Grieving. What's Wrong?
- Depression, Anxiety, & Fear
- Trauma & PTSD Side Effects No One Warned Me About
- Body Image & Sexuality: Seeing A Different Reflection
- The Importance of Mindfulness & Self-Care
- Who Am I?
- Is It Possible to Stay Positive?
- Feeling Overwhelmed: Is This the New Normal?
- Finding Your Way Through the Financial Fallout
- I'm Done with Treatment, So Now What?
- My Family: One Of the Effects I Didn't Know About
- Feelings of Isolation

***

Internet Research:

Staring Cancer in the Faith - Study Guide is the participant's guide that accompanies Project31's video curriculum. It includes 12 lessons learned along the journey after a diagnosis of breast cancer.

***

Today's Quote:

"The ultimate test of faith is not how loudly you praise God in happy times but how deeply you trust him in dark times."

—Rick Warren

A Note to You:

When I went to the class, each session was full of revelations. I confessed my deepest insecurities about faith and God. The leader said, "Take it to God. He already knows your innermost thoughts and feelings."

Those words felt so liberating! No matter what our spiritual beliefs may be, it's okay to seek clarity from our Divine Source. Hugs, my friend. We have a lot on our plates that others can't possibly understand.

Cancer Post #76: Today's Momentous Journey: September 21st

I underwent a biopsy of both my uterus and ovaries. It was an odd feeling; I was completely emotionless. Maybe this detachment enabled me to keep a level head.

At times like these, I'm so grateful for my breast cancer support groups. These women and men face the fear of another scan or biopsy with me. Jodi, a lady in my Livestrong Group, gave me a new tube of lipstick, a scarf, pink slippers, and a pink headband to let me know she cared. Sally gave me an inspiring poem. My sister sent me a funny card. My husband is always by my side. We fret before we get the results, yet the results may be splendid, and our apprehension was unnecessary.

***

Internet Research:

Adjustment to Cancer: Anxiety and Distress - NCI

Anxiety and distress can affect the quality of life of people with cancer and their families.

People living with cancer feel many different emotions, including anxiety and distress.

- Anxiety is unease, fear, and dread caused by stress.

- Distress is emotional, mental, social, or spiritual suffering. People who are distressed may have a range of feelings, from sadness and a loss of control to depression, anxiety, panic, and isolation.

***

Today's Quote:

"Anxiety is a lot like a toddler. It never stops talking, tells you you're wrong about everything, and wakes you up at 3 a.m."

—Anonymous

A Note to You:

I'm so grateful I have the support system I do. I know it isn't the same for everyone, and if you don't have that kind of support, please reach out to someone who can give you the encouragement and solidarity you need. You don't have to go through this journey alone, even if you feel shy. Find a group of survivors, and they'll wrap their arms around you in love and understanding. Each one of you reading this book is special and precious. While I understand that it's difficult, please try your best not to worry or be scared when scans, check-ups, or biopsies are scheduled. You have a whole Pink Sisterhood looking out for you and sending you strength.

Cancer Post #77: Weighing In: September 23rd

You may be wondering, why another post about weight? I've fought the scales since junior high, and it's been a long and difficult journey. On one hand, I want to be healthier and live a longer life. On the other hand, I am frustrated by the lack of progress and overwhelmed by how much I still have to lose. Somedays, it seems impossible to reach the desired weight my oncologist set for me, yet here I am, still struggling.

During one of my visits with my co-worker Courtnee, she expressed concern about my weight loss journey. She said, "I can see how hard you work to shed those extra pounds. With all the other challenges you're facing, it must be overwhelming to deal with this added stress." Her words were filled with empathy and compassion, and they truly touched my heart.

I explained to Courtnee my why.

"Courtnee," I said, "I truly appreciate you recognizing my determination to shed these pounds. My oncologist warned me that with the type of cancer I have and its aggressive nature, every extra ten pounds increases my risk of relapse by a whopping twenty percent. It's all because of the excess estrogen produced by fat in my body."

Courtnee's eyes widened in understanding, and she said, "You know I struggle with weight, too."

I continued. "Maybe we can mutually support each other?"

"Yes!" Courtnee replied.

"I don't want a recurrence, Courtnee," I said, "Even if that means giving up all the great treats people bring to work to share every day."

Here are the stats for yesterday. Did I want to scream about the gain? Yes. Consistency I keep telling myself. Well, at least I'm consistent about telling myself to be consistent.

PS... dig how many steps I walked. Even though the scales showed a gain I am so proud of the number of steps I got in.

Weight: Gain 1.8 pounds

Calories Consumed: 1552

Fit Bit Calories Out: 2,717

Steps: 19,467
Date Started: 08.11
Total pounds lost: 4.8
Today's Healthy Eating Tip:
I have faith in my willpower to succeed.

***

Internet Research:

Aromatase Inhibitor Treatment And Weight Gain | Food for Breast Cancer

Exercise appears to be the best strategy to prevent aromatase inhibitor-associated weight gain and body fat distribution changes. One study reported that a combined resistance and aerobic exercise program succeeded in improving body composition in breast cancer survivors taking aromatase inhibitors.

Today's Quote:

"Don't dig your grave with your own knife and fork."

—Author Unknown

A Note to You:

One of the biggest challenges I face while on a diet is saying no to unhealthy food made by well-meaning friends or family. They don't realize I have no control once I take a tiny bite. It's like a switch flips, and suddenly, I'm consumed with cravings for the entire cake, pie, or whatever it may be. If you deal with this same struggle, find an accountability partner who can help keep you from devouring the entire pizza!

Cancer Post #78: Passing the Torch: September 25th

My sister mailed me a pin to wear, a little brooch that she wore while undergoing cancer treatments. It's the famous pink ribbon symbol of breast cancer awareness, and I kept it close, wearing it in honor of my mother, my sister, and now me.

I saved this glittering pink ribbon pin just as my sister did. If another woman in our family develops breast cancer, I will pass it on to them. I hope I don't need to hand it down. I pray this disease ends with me. But if it doesn't, I hope this pin will give our courage and love to the next person needing it.

My friend Sally, another cancer survivor gave me a poem with a magnet on the back to hang on my refrigerator. She explained another survivor gave it to her, to remind her of strength and courage in the face of her own journey. "When the time comes that you feel someone else needs it more than you," Sally instructed, "pass it on."

***

Internet Research:

The Gift of Love

It matters much less what you choose to give as long as you give it with love.

***

Today's Quote:

"You don't have the power to make rainbows or waterfalls, sunsets or roses, but you do have the power to bless people by your words and smiles You carry within you the power to make the world better."

—Sharon G. Larsen

A Note to You:

Hold it close to your heart when you stumble upon something that eases your burdens, whether it's a trinket, a verse, or a story. And when the time comes, pass it on to another in need. For we are united in this journey called life.

Cancer Post #79: The Biopsy's Revelation: September 27th

My cell phone lit up at 4:30 p.m., and my heart raced as I slid my finger across the screen to answer. My mouth went dry, and sweat beaded on my forehead as I waited for a voice on the other end. The biopsy results could either push me between ultimate joy or unimaginable sorrow.

I was beyond confused as I talked to the nurse. "I see you called asking about your lab results?" she said in a strange, almost accusatory tone.

"Yes," I said.

"What results are you calling about?" she asked.

"The results of the biopsy I had on Wednesday," I replied.

The nurse's voice fell silent. Then she asked, "So you haven't spoken to the doctor yet?"

"The doctor never called me," I blurted out in fear.

The nurse went quiet momentarily, but I didn't let the silence drag on. "Can you tell me, is the mass benign or malignant?" I asked.

"It's normal," she said. Again silence.

"That's good, right?" I asked.

"Yes," she said.

As soon as the call ended, I felt relief wash over me. The news that I didn't have ovarian cancer filled me with joy. Despite this, I couldn't help but feel confused about the phone call. Why had the nurse been so secretive? And why didn't they inform me beforehand on Friday, saving me from worrying all weekend?

After I sighed in relief, a quirky thought came to my head. Did this nurse understand what she was looking at during our conversation?

The next day, I called the doctor's office and asked for a copy of my report because I couldn't find it on my patient portal. Despite the nurse's reassurance that the results were normal, something about her tone felt off—could it have been her mood that day?

Internet Research:

How to Ask for Clarification (voanews.com)

Express lack of understanding

The first step is to tell the person that you are not sure that you have understood them fully.

• I'm sorry, but I'm not sure (that) I understand.

• Sorry, I'm not sure (that) I know what you mean.

• Sorry but I don't quite follow you.

After you express your lack of understanding, the next step is to ask the person to clarify what they have said. Here are some phrases you can use.

• Could you say it in another way?

• Can you clarify that for me?

• Could you rephrase that?

Other times, you may simply need more information or a helpful example. In such situations, the following are useful:

• Could you be more specific?

• Can you give me an example?

• Could you elaborate on that?

Offer thanks

After the person clarifies themselves, you can let them know that you now understand and are thankful.

***

Today's Quote:

"The two words 'information' and 'communication' are often used interchangeably, but they signify quite different things. Information is giving out; communication is getting through."

—Sydney J. Harris

A Note to You:

Today's cancer research was a real eye-opener for me. These communication tips are game-changing. I wrote them down on a sticky note and stuck them on my computer screen. Next time you're having one of those intense chats, following these suggestions will make things go much smoother. There will be no more frustration, just good vibes.

Cancer Post #80: The Doctor's Call: September 28th

I decided to be brave and once again call the doctor's office. I wasn't entirely confident about what the nurse said about my lab results. Unless I felt certain, there was no way I could settle down regarding my potential diagnosis of cancer. Thus, I would persist until I got a sense of relief.

    The doctor called me back, her voice comforting and reassuring as she reported the tumors were benign. I allowed myself to truly relax for the first time since the initial phone call left me with a nagging question in my head.

    I couldn't wait to tell my Livestrong community that the growth in my body wasn't cancerous. I sent a short message to everyone in the group. Arriving at the gym that evening, my friends stood up and cheered for me when I entered our meeting room. I cried happy tears.

    Studies say you can't feel out of the woods until you have been cancer-free for five years. But I defy this warning, feeling as though the menacing presence of the disease has relinquished its hold, and I have been swept away to a highway where I can travel freely. No more dark woods with unknown entities lurking in wait, only a clear path towards my future - Cancer-free.

***

Internet Research:

5-year cancer survival rate: Can cancer patient only live for 5 years? (medicaltrend.org)

Many people will ask why we should choose a 5-year survival rate instead of a 1-year, 2-year survival rate. This is because the peak period of cancer recurrence and metastasis is the first 5 years after surgery. If there is no recurrence or metastasis within 5 years, the probability of recurrence and metastasis is very low, and it can be considered that a clinical cure has been achieved.

***

Today's Quote:

"Being assertive does not mean attacking or ignoring other's feelings. It means that you are willing to hold up for yourself fairly-without attacking others."

—Albert Ellis

A Note for You:

As someone who has been through cancer and knows the struggles of mental and physical illness, I want you to know that it's okay to ask questions. You are brave and resilient and never hesitate to seek answers until you feel empowered and informed.

SHELLEY MALICOTE STUTCHMAN

NOTES AND THOUGHTS

Chapter Twenty-Six

BODY REMODELING

Cancer Post #81: Breast Size: October 5th

As I prepared for my body remodeling, I felt excited. With the help of my excellent plastic surgeon and newfound energy, my desire for transformation was fueled. I realized I could use the same creativity I used for rearranging furniture and decorating for the holidays to shape and mold my body. After all, my physical self is my living space.

I eagerly entered the plastic surgeon's office. After meeting all the out-of-pocket deductibles, my body remodel job felt like getting free plastic surgery! The chance for a complete transformation had me buzzing with anticipation and joy.

At the age of fifty, I underwent a procedure for breast implants. While having tests on my breasts, doctors discovered a leak in the implant in my non-cancerous side. Thankfully, I qualified for insurance coverage to have both breasts redone. My surgeon said by doing both breasts, I would look symmetrical once again.

I faced a tough choice: maintain my current size, increase it, or decrease it. I eliminated the option of going bigger. I considered going a bit smaller. I debated if the new position of my breasts, being more upright and higher on my chest, might look strange on someone my age.

I tugged my shirt up a bit to peer at my chest in the mirror. I sighed. If I went smaller and they were perky, I couldn't help but wonder if that would make me look thinner and younger. Then, on the other hand, I questioned, would I be disappointed if I reduced the size since seventeen years ago, I spent money to make my breasts fuller and larger? Oh, the decisions! For a change, these were fun choices.

I struggled with the decision of what breast size to choose. I weighed the pros and cons of different sizes and debated for hours.

Here is something I learned:

The most attractive breast size is between a C and a D cup, but firmness and pertness are more attractive than size.

That information completely bewildered me. Size C was supposedly the most attractive, yet I wanted that oh-so-desired perky look. Not sure what to do or what would be best for my body, I decided to pay my surgeon a visit. Maybe she could help me make sense of it all.

***

Internet Research:

https://blackdoctor.org/breast-implants-risks

The larger your implant, the worse your breast will look over time. A larger implant will stretch your tissues over time and will cause more tissue-thinning and sagging than a smaller implant. Your tissues do not improve with age, and they will be less able to support the additional weight of any implant, especially a larger implant.

***

Today's Quote:

"Okay, let's see if I got this straight. The butt is the new breast, and the lower back is the new ankle. Now if only we could figure out where the brain has moved."

—Celia Rivenbark

A Note for You:

When it comes to breast reconstruction after cancer, you need to understand that it's not about vanity. It's about moving forward. You have the choice to go flat or undergo reconstruction, and either way, it's your decision. For me personally, breast reconstruction was a fun opportunity to remodel my chest and take back control of my body. So, if you do decide to have reconstruction, don't stress about things like breast size. Instead, embrace the chance to go on a fun breast-shopping spree! Remember that this is a time to celebrate your strength and resilience in overcoming cancer.

Cancer Post #82: A Deceased Woman's Breast: October 8th

During my consultation with the plastic surgeon, we discussed the size and shape of my new breasts. After browsing countless articles on the internet, I finally decided and told her, "I prefer a more modest size with a perky appearance." Then, I explained to her, "It might be best to choose an implant that is smaller in size as my skin ages since it will hold up better over time."

The plastic surgeon pulled her digital notebook from her bag and scribbled notes on the screen. "We can do that, but it will be more complicated. You will have sagging skin and need to come back for a second surgery. It will be a one-step procedure if you stay the same size."

I did not want more surgery than necessary, so I answered, "Then let's go for the same size."

The surgeon gave me a detailed overview of the upcoming procedure, adding it would be sometime in November. She informed me that I would need to take two weeks away from work and avoid any heavy exercise or lifting for four weeks post-surgery.

She said due to the size of the cavity in my breast, she may need to fill it with tissue taken from a cadaver - instead of implants like I had expected.

As I heard the surgeon explain about reconstructing my body with the tissue of someone who is no longer living, I was filled with a mix of emotions. A profound admiration for the remarkable generosity of a total stranger, combined with tremendous guilt at being the sole recipient of such kindness. My mind raced with thoughts as I imagined having a lifelong connection to this person whom I would never be able to thank face to face.

I am immensely grateful to those who checked the box for organ and tissue donation. Your selfless act of kindness has saved so many lives. If I end up using the skin and tissue of a donor, I would love to thank the family for bringing up such a big-hearted person. I played it forward by donating any parts of my body to use in helping others when I die. It would be an honor to follow in the footsteps of the person willing to share with me if needed.

Generously donated tissue is one of many options available for breast reconstruction surgery, and one tissue donor can help up to ten breast reconstruction patients.

***

Internet Research:

Alloderm Regenerative Tissue Matrix | RealSelf

AlloDerm is a material derived from donated human skin that's placed in the body to reinforce tissue and provide a foundation for regeneration. It was originally developed in 1994 as a graft for burn patients, and its pliable, versatile nature makes it useful for many plastic surgery procedures, including facial reconstruction, abdominal wall reconstruction, and breast reconstruction.

"It consists of the deeper skin layer, with all of the cells removed, so it is essentially a sheet of collagen," says Dr. Richard Baxter, a plastic surgeon in Mountlake Terrace, Washington, in a RealSelf Q&A. "The body recognizes it as 'self' and sends in your own cells to populate the graft, along with blood vessels, and so on."

An AlloDerm graft is most often used in implant-based breast reconstruction surgeries, for added support. "After a pocket has been created for the expander or implant following a mastectomy, AlloDerm is placed inside the pocket and stitched into the chest wall, to keep it in place," explains Dr. Morgan Norris, a Houston-based plastic surgeon, in a RealSelf Q&A. "Once it is secured, the AlloDerm acts as reinforcement. It also helps the body stabilize the implant and reduces implant migration."

***

Today's Quote:

"The decision to be an organ donor is the embodiment of faith in the power of humanity to heal, to save and to prevail."

—Unknown

A Note to You:

My plastic surgeon opened my eyes to the life-saving impact of organ donation, and it really made me think. If you're capable and willing, please consider signing up as a donor. Even if you can't donate organs due to your cancer history, there are still other tissues like skin or corneas that could save someone's life. Just think about the incredible difference you could make for someone else, another woman like us, who deserves a second chance at life.

NOTES AND THOUGHTS

Chapter Twenty-Seven

ANXIETY TRIGGERS

Cancer Post #83: Well, This is Scary: October 9th

Understanding the statistics related to breast cancer is crucial. As someone who has always been intrigued by numbers, I found the statistics surrounding breast cancer particularly interesting. Here are a few noteworthy statistics that shed light on the impact of breast cancer on women's health.

***

Internet Research:

Breast Cancer by State: Comparing Mortality Rates Across the U.S. (nationalbreastcancer.org)

Based on nationwide breast cancer incidence and death (mortality) rates provided by the CDC, the following information can be inferred:

Rhode Island has the highest breast cancer incidence rate in the country. Hawaii has the highest screening rate in the country.

- Hawaii has the highest breast cancer survival rate.

- California has the highest number of new breast cancer cases in the country.

- California has the highest number of breast cancer deaths.

- The most common type of breast cancer is Invasive Ductal Carcinoma (IDC). IDC makes up about 70-80% of all breast cancers.

***

Today's Quote:

"Medicine is a science of uncertainty and an art of probability."

—William Osler

A Note to You:

My fellow pink sisters, have you ever considered how we are statistics in the realm of breast cancer? We never wanted to be part of these numbers, but by being here, we offer valuable information for public health planning and awareness. Our stories and experiences as survivors matter so much.

Cancer Post #84: Rash: October 11th

October tenth marked the fourth month since I declared myself cancer-free. We celebrated by going out for a lovely shrimp dinner at Red Lobster and sharing pink ribbon cookies with our friends at Staring Cancer in the Faith.

I also had a six-month check-up with the surgeon who removed the tumor. With her skilled hands, she carefully checked each breast for any abnormalities. She explained there was a build-up of scar tissue where they inserted the Brachytherapy bulb. I needed to massage this area daily. Then she laughed and said, "I am not talking about a light massage with lotion. Massage that area until it almost hurts you are pressing so hard."

"Great," I thought, "That sounded pleasant."

The surgeon uncrossed her arms and leaned forward in her chair, a patient look of understanding on her face. "I'd like you to come back and see me every six months for the next five years," she said. I wondered why I was being asked to keep coming back so often. Nodding slowly, I made a mental note not to forget to ask before my appointment in March why so often.

I pointed to the bright red rash that had developed on my neck a few weeks prior. The plastic surgeon had prescribed a steroid cream, but I was still fearful of what it may have been. When my doctor looked at the rash, she told me something I never expected: there could be a link between rashes and breast cancer. I wanted to share this information with others who may not know about this possible connection.

She peered at me and said soberly, "I am not concerned with the rash on your neck. But if you spot any rashes, bumps, or anything else on your chest, please call my office and come in. A chest rash can be a sign of breast cancer."

That was the first I had ever heard about rashes on the chest as a sign of breast cancer. So, I Googled it, and here is what I found in my research:

Internet Research:

What a Breast Cancer Rash Is, and How to Tell If You Have One - Parade: Entertainment, Recipes, Health, Life, Holidays

When it comes to red flags around breast cancer, most women know that feeling a new lump in your breast is a reason to seek medical attention immediately. But as it turns out, a rash is also something to be mindful of. This is due to the fact that some breast cancers are inflammatory and manifest in the form of a breast cancer rash.

"When we think about skin changes associated with breast cancer it could be because the cancer is either invading or growing through the skin or inflammatory breast cancer," Dr. Michele Ley, MD, FACS, a breast surgical oncologist at Arizona Oncology, explains. "There are other skin conditions that can occur on the breast just as they can occur elsewhere in the body like psoriasis, eczema, or dermatitis."

"Inflammatory breast cancer is a rare, but serious form of breast cancer that can present as a rash with or without breast swelling and a breast mass," says Dr. Mitchell Gross, Associate Professor of Clinical Medicine at the Keck School of Medicine of USC and the Research Director of the Lawrence J. Ellison Institute for Transformative Medicine.

If a woman is concerned about a rash on the breast, she should get evaluated by a medical professional immediately.

***

Today's Quote:

"Learning is the beginning of wealth. Learning is the beginning of health. Learning is the beginning of spirituality. Searching and learning is where the miracle process all begins."

—Jim Rohn

A Note to You:

As members of the pink sisterhood, we must remain vigilant and aware of any changes in or on our bodies now that we have experienced breast cancer. I'm not trying to scare you, but rather to potentially save you. Who would have thought that a seemingly harmless rash could actually be another indication of breast cancer?

Cancer Post #85: Swimming Suit Anxiety: October 16th

In the following posts, we will take a closer look at the mental and emotional aspects of Breast Cancer. This is something often overlooked by those who are providing medical care for someone diagnosed with cancer. However, I believe paying attention to the psychological is just as important.

Thursday evening, we gathered for our Livestrong program, and discussed our upcoming water aerobics class. The doctor instructed me to stay out of swimming pools and hot tubs all summer, but I no longer had that excuse. I was free to be a mermaid. My worry may sound dumb, but I was scared to death to put on a swimsuit. Due to surgeries, scars crisscrossed my breast like decorative stitching on a quilt.

My fingers wandered hesitantly over my chest, tracing thirty-six tiny scars left behind by the radiation therapy. My partial mastectomy incision healed well, but the disfigurement underneath my arm from where they removed my lymph nodes was still visible. Anxiety stirred inside me as I realized none of my swimsuits would cover the scars.

I wanted to try water aerobics. Then I remembered my bonus daughter Melissa showed me some long-sleeve swimsuits online. I checked them out and thought they were cute. Thanks to my buddy Amazon, I found a bright yellow and black suit. True to form, Amazon had it at my door in just a few days. It covered me up like a nun.

When I walked into the class in my new swimsuit, I felt nervous and excited. My sister had come to spend the night with me and borrowed one of my sexier swimsuits. As I looked at her in admiration, I was envious of her. She was a cancer survivor with a beautiful tattoo covering her scars. Her courage made me wonder if she had felt the same anxiety as I did when it came to putting her body on display in a swimsuit for the first time after surgery.

I entered the pool area, elated to find it reserved for our particular group of survivors. I dipped my toe into the cool water before taking the plunge with a splash. As I surfaced and looked around, I noticed the ladies' swimsuits ranged from simple T-shirts worn over their suits to modest and even revealing daring, sexy swimwear. Some of the ladies already had their reconstruction, some had chosen to remain flat, and there was me waiting for my implants. In this moment of togetherness, every woman in the pool radiated impressive beauty.

The instructor cranked up the speakers and played upbeat music. We were instantly entranced and splashed around in a synchronized frenzy. Everyone grinned from ear to ear as we swayed our hips, exercised, and laughed. It was an absolute riot!

My body was slick with water and chlorine as I finished my swim class. I tugged at the damp fabric of my long-sleeved swimsuit, struggling to peel it off my skin. It fit perfectly when dry, but now it clung stubbornly to me. But you know what? The next time I went swimming, I wore one of my old swimsuits with colorful stripes that always made me feel confident and empowered. I proudly displayed the scars on my body from my battle with cancer. I am a survivor and refuse to be held back by a stubborn swimsuit.

***

Internet Research:

6 Swimsuit Brands for Breast Cancer Thrivers! - Rethink Breast Cancer

Wearing a swimsuit can already be an unsettling experience for many women. Wearing a swimsuit post-mastectomy or lumpectomy? Try quadrupling that self-consciousness. But, at Rethink, we see breast cancer thrivers as beautiful, courageous, amazing women who deserve to enjoy their fun in the sun. Period.

***

Today's Quote:

"I always say, 'Do you have a body? Then you're swimsuit ready.' That's all you need to worry about."

—Emily Ratajkowski

A Note to You:

As a fellow survivor, I know when it comes to wearing swimsuits, we may feel anxious and insecure about our bodies. But let me tell you this: don't let the scars keep you away from the swimming pool if that is your passion. Specialized swimsuits for breast cancer patients are available online or in physical stores. And if you are too conscious about your scars, why not follow my sister's example: get a beautiful or fun tattoo to cover them up? Let nothing stop you from enjoying life.

SHELLEY MALICOTE STUTCHMAN

NOTES AND THOUGHTS

Chapter Twenty-Eight
GHOSTING

Cancer Post #86: Vanishing Act: October 27th

I was ghosted. It hurt. I read on cancer websites that ghosting is real for many cancer patients and survivors. I am not talking about seeing ghosts in white sheets. I am talking about friends and family who suddenly ignore you.

I'm forever thankful for the encouragement I received from my family, friends, and Facebook circle, as well as all the new connections that I made because of cancer. Unfortunately, some of my previous friends just weren't there for me. It stings; when you're dealing with a serious illness like cancer, something as simple as a text message or card from your pals can make a world of difference in your day.

I educated myself on cancer ghosting. Most articles said it happens because the person does not know what to say or is afraid of saying the wrong thing and feels terrible about it later. I wondered if the real truth this happens is because the old friend may be worried you will ask them to run an errand or some other tasks you need help accomplishing while you are ill. However, articles I read recommend that you go easy on your friends because it is hard for them to think of you as sick, and they can't deal with the idea you may die from your illness.

If you have been ghosted, copy this paragraph and send it to the friend who ghosted you. If you have ghosted a friend or family member and are reading this, forget about your lame excuses. Do the right thing and take a minute to send a text. You'll make the recipient's day with that gesture. If you are worried about what to talk about, remember your friend is still the same person. Your friend may want to hear how you are doing and what is taking place in your life as well.

***

Internet Research:

Cancer Ghosting: When Friends Can't Deal with a Diagnosis| SurvivorNet

It's hardly surprising that some people become tongue-tied when speaking with cancer survivors, worried they'll say the wrong thing or not offer the needed comfort or support. But what might come as a surprise is the amount of survivors who say that people they were close to stopped speaking to them altogether after they were diagnosed.

"Ghosting" — or the process of cutting ties with someone suddenly and with no explanation — is apparently prevalent in the cancer community.

Informal research conducted by War on Cancer, a social networking app for survivors, found that 65% of surveyed survivors said they had friends or relatives who cut contact or pulled away from them after they were diagnosed.

***

Today's Quote:

"Friends can help each other. A true friend is someone who lets you have total freedom to be yourself – and especially to feel. Or not feel. Whatever you happen to be feeling at the moment is fine with them. That's what real love amounts to – letting a person be what he really is."

—Jim Morrison

A Note to You:

I know how much it hurts to be ghosted, especially during this time when we need our loved ones the most. I went through it, too, and I regret not confronting those who left me. But I learned a valuable lesson. Don't be afraid to confront those who ghosted you. Maybe things could've been different if I had, but I never took that chance. If it's someone close, why not message and tell that person how much you miss him or her? If you receive no reply, that person was never a good friend. But if you receive a kind response, your friendship can be mended. Sending you hugs, my dear friend.

… SHELLEY MALICOTE STUTCHMAN

NOTES AND THOUGHTS

Chapter Twenty-Nine

FOGGY BRAIN

Cancer Post #87: Echoes of Forgetfulness: November 6th

At my follow-up with the radiologist, I inquired, "I understand that you like seeing me, but I am unsure of the purpose of this appointment. Could you please enlighten me?"

"Your body has been through a tumultuous journey. I need to check on the healing process of the scars left by the insertion of the tubes," the radiologist explained.

"Is this my final visit with you?" I asked.

She let out a small laugh, "I know it would be nice to just have one visit and be done, but with cancer, we need to closely monitor you for five years. You'll continue seeing your entire team regularly." She reached out and placed a comforting hand on my shoulder before continuing. "You'll see me again in six months, and then, if everything looks good, we'll move to annual check-ups for the next five years."

My radiologist's brutal honesty gave me a strong sense of trust in her and the fact she treated me as an equal. Her statements cut through the sugar-coated words of others, piercing straight to the heart of my condition.

"How have you been holding up?" she inquired after completing the examination.

"I have some things I'm worried about. But I think they are side effects of the Letrozole. I guess I should keep those questions for my oncologist," I responded.

She spun her small doctor's stool to face me. I could tell by the way she gazed at me she was ready for me to share my concerns. Perhaps my unease was visible in my expression.

"Something is wrong," I blurted out, unable to contain the worry that had been building inside me. "The hot flashes are coming more frequently now, leaving me drenched in sweat. And the joint pain, once manageable, is now becoming unbearable, making it difficult to move or even sleep."

"Go on," she coaxed.

"I'm afraid the medication is starting to affect my mind," I said. I placed my hand on my forehead, feeling a slight headache and confusion settling in. "Or maybe it's something more serious. I can't shake off this fear of dementia creeping in."

"What makes you think that?" she asked.

"My mind has become a jumbled mess of scattered thoughts and forgetfulness. Everything slips through the cracks no matter how hard I try to keep track. I wanted to donate canned goods for the food drive at work, but it was already over by the time I remembered. And when your nurse asked for my gynecologist's name, I drew a complete blank. It's frustrating not being able to rely on my memory anymore."

Now there was no stopping me. "Sometimes my words stumble out of my mouth like a drunkard, slurring into incoherent messes. Last week, in front of the group at Livestrong, I tried to say that Jodi would be providing most of the food. Instead, I said, Jodi will provide most of the money. The room erupted in laughter, but I felt like a clown with a painted-on smile covering my embarrassment."

I continued, "My husband and I were watching the news, but my thoughts were jumbled. Suddenly, I blurted out, "Is Hillary going to win?"

I remember my mind was racing, trying to decide if she was even running for president. My husband gave me a confused look, probably wondering what was going through my head.

I confided to my radiologist, "I'm scared. The constant joint pain, waves of nausea, fatigue, and hot flashes are bad. But what truly frightens me is the thought of losing my ability to think. I pride myself on my sharp mind. The cognitive decline terrifies me."

My doctor answered, "You don't have dementia. Let me explain what is happening."

She took a deep breath before continuing, "You were taking hormone replacement therapy when you received your diagnosis. As per your oncologist's instructions, you stopped taking the hormones and started on Letrozole. Your hormones and brain are closely linked, and hormonal changes can affect memory."

I kept quiet, pondering her connection of the hormones to brain comment.

"I've seen it happen before," she said with a knowing look. "Women who were on HRT, then given a hormone blocker, sometimes have the worst side effects."

Inhaling deeply, I couldn't help but feel grateful. I wasn't losing my mind. I looked at my life and everything I still had to do: writing a book, maintaining a job, and loving my family. This medication was supposed to save me, but it felt like it was slowly killing me instead.

After my appointment, I joined Jeanne at Whiskey Cake for dinner. Each step felt like a hammer striking my knees, and I fought to climb the curb. Always perceptive and compassionate, Jeanne noticed my struggle and wordlessly grasped my hand, steadying me as I stumbled. After our meal, we headed to her new house, where she once again provided physical support as we ascended the porch steps. The side effects of Letrozole put me at risk of sustaining severe injuries from even a minor fall, a cruel reminder this medication weakened me while fighting cancer within my body.

Throughout the weekend, I debated whether to stop taking the medication or request a different brand from my oncologist. My research revealed that, without a hormone blocker, my type of cancer had a higher chance of returning.

As I researched the different hormone blocker options, I grew disheartened by the fact that Letrozole remained the top choice. It all boiled down to money - insurance companies prioritizing the cheapest option, regardless of its potential side effects. They couldn't possibly understand the excruciating agony I endured in bed, pleading for relief from the unrelenting pain caused by this medication chosen solely for its cost. This harsh reality fueled my anger and broke my heart.

I discovered a Facebook support group for women on Letrozole and other hormone blockers. I'm grateful for Facebook groups. The name of the group is" Anastrozole, Letrozole, Exemestane, and Tamoxifen...Living with Side Effects."

I found out from a Facebook group that some oncologists will wean their patients off of their HRT for eight weeks before starting hormone blockers. This gradual transition helps the body adjust instead of suddenly stopping HRT and starting blocker medication. It's a sensible approach that I wish I had been given as an option during my transition.

Frustrated and desperate, I phoned my oncologist's office. I requested the nurse to get the doctor to change my medication. I waited anxiously for a callback. I longed to feel like myself again - vibrant, energetic, and alive. But as days passed with no return call, I decided to take matters into my own hands.

***

Internet Research:

https://www.pacificneuroscienceinstitute.org/

Hormones and memory loss

In women, estrogen regulates cortisol, a neurotransmitter responsible for chemical communications in the brain. Estrogen levels decline over time, especially during peri-menopause, and cortisol levels in the brain are not well regulated. What causes memory loss is this breakdown of chemical signaling. While this is a natural process of aging, women often report symptoms of depression, fatigue and insomnia.

***

Today's Quote:

"Here's to the crazy ones. The misfits. The rebels. The troublemakers. The round pegs in the square holes. The ones who see things differently. They're not fond of rules. And they have no respect for the status quo. You can quote them, disagree with them, glorify or vilify them. About the only thing you can't do is ignore them. Because they change things. They push the human race forward. And while some may see them as the crazy ones, we see genius. Because the people who are crazy enough to think they can change the world, are the ones who do."

—Rob Siltanen

A Note to You:

Hey, I hope everything's going well with your hormone blocker. Those side effects can be rough, huh? I totally get it. The brain fog was the worst for me. It's so frustrating not being able to remember stuff. It felt like I was disappearing and being replaced by someone else. Like, who am I becoming? But seriously, if you're feeling any side effects from these drugs, talk to your oncologist. Don't let your doctors brush you off. They need to take your concerns seriously. And if they don't, it might be time to find a new doctor who will listen to you. Losing our sharp minds is definitely one of the hardest parts of dealing with cancer, but guess what? We're fighters, and we will win this battle! Sending you lots of love and hugs, my friend.

Cancer Post #88: Try to Remember: November 9th

I reached out to my oncologist after a few days. Enduring the joint pain, weight fluctuations, bloating, and nausea caused by the cancer medication proved to be a challenge. But the memory loss terrified me. I treasured my ability to think clearly. I adamantly refused to let the hormone blocker rob me of my cognitive abilities; I would rather face death than lose my capacity for rational thought.

After much deliberation, I decided to take a break from Letrozole for two weeks in the hopes of easing the overwhelming side effects. The tiny yellow pill had wreaked havoc on my body and mind, and I was eager for some relief. According to my research, most of its effects would subside within a week or so after stopping the medication. While trying to stay positive, the fear of cancer returning lingered in the back of my mind. But I weighed the risks and prioritized my cognitive abilities over losing brain power due to this medication. I also reached out to my team at work, asking for their understanding and patience as I may not be functioning at my usual level.

After enduring months of unbearable side effects, my doctor and I decided to try another brand of hormone blocker. Little did I know that the new medication was significantly more expensive than the one that caused me so much suffering.

The doctor prescribed Exemestane or Aromasin. But as I read about its possible side effects—hot flashes, insomnia, weight gain, hair loss—I couldn't help but question the risk. She thought the new drug might have less impact on my cognitive function, which I saw as a significant benefit. Wigs were an option if my hair fell out, but I only had one brain. The decision weighed heavily on my thought process. This thought crossed my mind many times: we don't fight and win against cancer to continue suffering.

Internet Research:

https://www.webmd.com/drugs/2/drug-17764/exemestane

Remember that this medication has been prescribed because your doctor has judged that the benefit to you is greater than the risk of side effects.

***

Today's Quote:

"Knowledge is the life of the mind."

—Abu Bakr As-Siddiq (RA)

A Note to You:

I understand the pain you must be going through as cancer takes its toll. The constant rounds of treatment feel never-ending, and the fear of losing yourself is overwhelming. With determination and the support of skilled doctors, victory is within your reach. Let these words be a comforting hug during this challenging fight. Your pink sisters are here beside you every step of the way.

Cancer Post #89: Skin Cancer Side Effect: November 13th

Another doctor's visit, different office, different doctor, same sterile, white-washed walls. As my dermatologist finished his examination of my skin, I felt tense. Before the breast cancer diagnosis the past few years have brought me a skin cancer scare and in-office procedures to remove those cancers. Finally, the doctor gave me the all-clear for another year. With a sigh of relief, I mustered up the courage to ask the question that had been weighing heavily on my mind: "Now that I've battled breast cancer, am I at a higher risk for skin cancer?"

"It depends," he said.

I thought, here we go again, another one of those, it depends' answers that doctors usually give.

Fortunately, he redeemed himself and proceeded to enlighten me on the fact that individuals who have undergone radiation therapy are at a higher risk of developing skin cancer in the treated area. Since skin cancer can manifest many years after treatment, monitoring your skin and seeking advice from a dermatologist is even more critical.

***

Internet Research:

The Surprising Link Between Breast Cancer and Skin Cancer | Water's Edge Dermatology (wederm.com)

Anyone who's had breast cancer or skin cancer should know the unfortunate truth: Having one of these diseases seems to increase the likelihood of developing the other.

In a 2011 study, female breast cancer survivors under age 45 had a 38% increased risk for developing melanoma compared to the general population. Among women over 45 who survived breast cancer, the increased risk for melanoma was 12%.

A 2013 study found that women (average age 66) who'd had non-melanoma skin cancer had a 19% increased risk for eventually being diagnosed with breast cancer. A study of more than 70,000 postmenopausal women published the same year found no link between non-melanoma skin cancers and breast cancer — but it discovered that women with a history of basal cell or squamous cell cancer who developed breast cancer were more likely to have an advanced case of breast cancer.

***

Today's Quote:

"What is your skin trying to tell you? Often the skin is a metaphor for deeper issues and a way for your body to send up a red flag to warn you that all is not well underneath."

—Dr. Judyth Reichenberg

A Note for You:

I understand the frustration and fear you may be feeling about the increased risk of skin cancer as a result of breast cancer. It's overwhelming, but knowledge is power. We can't bury our heads in the sand - we must face it head-on. By being aware and vigilant, we can take steps to protect ourselves and stay prepared for whatever comes our way. Don't let this news discourage you. Use it as motivation to fight even harder against this disease.

Cancer Post #90: Echoes of Kinship: November 18th

As Thanksgiving approached, I reflected on an unexpected blessing that cancer brought into my life. Despite the hardship and struggle it caused, cancer also gave me something extraordinary - my tribe. Without this illness, I may have never crossed paths with the Livestrong program, which led me to a diverse and supportive group of men and women. Each of them became an integral part of my life, and I can't imagine where I'd be without their love and companionship. Cancer may have taken a lot from me, but it also gave me a precious gift of their friendship.

Every Tuesday and Thursday evening, a small group of cancer survivors and their support persons gathered at the local YMCA. As mentioned in a past post, the program, known as Livestrong, offers free workouts to help regain strength and also includes a one-year membership to the facility. When I joined the group, I had no idea I would end up finding my tribe within its walls.

Our last meeting felt bittersweet as we gathered for a Friendsgiving celebration and certificate presentation. We watched each person receive a letter of completion and heard progress scores. Our scores showed our incredible physical growth, but the emotional support we received couldn't be measured. I wanted to reflect on each group member to give you a feel of what you may find if you join this program.

Cameron: Our charismatic leader commanded our attention as he led us through stretches, cardio routines, and weight machines. He pushed us to our limits with a sweet smile, understanding our struggles yet never letting us quit. With each victory, no matter how small, Cameron celebrated us like champions, stealing our hearts and molding us into unstoppable machines of strength and endurance.

Garrett: Our assistant leader shared his life stories with us and listened intensely when we shared our struggles or tears. Garrett loved to research and find answers to our questions. We will carry Garrett's affection for us in our hearts forever.

Jodi: Our fearless leader. She was and continues to be a gentle and nurturing mother to us, always ensuring we had everything we needed. Whether sending encouraging texts before surgeries or medical tests or organizing Taco Tuesday after class, Jodi was always there for us. She exuded warmth and love, creating a sense of family within our group. And on those Tuesday nights at Yo Pablo's, when we gathered for $2 tacos and beers, it felt like a true fellowship. But Jodi's generosity went beyond just her time and efforts - she showered us with cancer swag items and mouth-watering snacks during the twelve weeks. It was no surprise when I saw a trophy in her home during our Friendsgiving celebration and learned a few years earlier she had received the Woman of Inspiration award. That award perfectly encapsulated Jodi - selfless, inspiring, and deserving of recognition.

Gary: Jodi's devoted husband and unshakeable support system graced us with his presence at each of our workouts. His muscular frame and unwavering presence inspired the group on the rewards of consistent healthy habits. Gary not only understood the struggles we girls faced, but he also welcomed and actively participated in our intimate conversations. Alongside Jodi, he was the perfect host as we gathered for a warm and inviting Friendsgiving in their home. And let me tell you, the ribs Gary cooked will forever be etched in my memory - they were simply divine, an exquisite blend of flavors and tender meat I know I'll never taste the likes of again until he makes his next batch.

Sally: She is synonymous with sunshine. Her dazzling smile brightens up every room she enters. Her God-given gift is making everyone feel at ease and accepted. Sally is my personal hero. During her youth, she embarked on a solo backpacking trip through Europe, displaying the courage I wish I possessed. Sally was always there whenever we needed a pillar of strength to lean on.

Doyle: Sally's sweet husband and support system, a gentleman with a soft-spoken demeanor. Doyle fought for us as a young man serving our country and stood by us as cancer survivors. He encouraged everyone in the group, pushing himself and exercising alongside us as we worked towards regaining our strength. We found joy in cheering Doyle on as he progressed, his body becoming more flexible and stronger. Every time we clapped or cheered for Doyle, a warm smile spread across his face, and his eyes lit up, filling us with warmth and camaraderie.

Lynette: Lynette wore T-shirts to each class with pictures and logos displaying cancer survivor slogans or designs. She encouraged us to embrace our survival and wear it as a badge of honor. Her infectious enthusiasm inspired us to do the same. During one of our Taco Tuesday gatherings, Lynette's cell phone rang, and we jumped at the sound of meowing coming from her purse. It turns out Lynette used to own exotic cats and loved to tell about them. We all looked forward to talking with Lynette because she had such an adventurous life and always had new stories. Whenever I'm out in the community, I know Lynette is nearby when I see her bright yellow sports car zooming around. The color perfectly matches her vibrant personality. She is genuine and authentic, and you can feel her love without her even saying a word.

Rene: She added sparkle to our group. Her contagious energy, adorable giggle, and creative ideas always cheered us. Rene was a great problem solver. She noticed we needed help with where to put our phones and purses during our workout sessions. So, at one of our meetings, Rene surprised each of the ladies with a personalized handmade bag that held all our essentials. Now, we all have a unique Rene design that hangs around our necks and under our arms, freeing up our hands for exercise. Rene's presence made our workouts more fun and enjoyable.

Dave: Rene's husband and support person. Dave is a man I truly admire. Despite needing a portable oxygen tank, Dave never missed our exercise classes. He encouraged and pushed us to do our best. Watching him persevere through his own challenges inspired us to keep going. Dave never showed any signs of self-pity or complained about his situation. Instead, he motivated us all to never give up, and to reach our goals. Dave exercised with dedication and determination, becoming a shining example and inspiration to all of us.

Jackie: She was our cheerleader; her excitement was evident in how she bounced and clapped her hands with every small victory we achieved. I later discovered that in high school, she had been a member of the cheerleading squad - a fact that made perfect sense to me. Jackie was cute, spunky, and funny. One of her bucket list goals was to do improv.

I hope she does because her tribe will be on the front row. During one of our classes, Jackie shared a new term for an ex-husband - a wasbund. Translation...he was your husband. It was the perfect blend of humor and truth, and I couldn't help but adopt the term myself. Jackie is one of those naturally funny people who keeps you rolling. I can always think of something funny about six hours later, but Jackie's quick wit kept the class in stitches. The good kind of stitches, that is.

Susan: She was Jackie's support person. Susan and Jackie showed us by example what true friendship is all about. Susan bore her own hardships but always managed to smile on and push through the tasks. Susan listened with open ears and a compassionate heart whenever our group gathered for support. She truly embodied what it meant to be a friend."

Neil: Cameraman, as people like to call him, has always been my biggest fan. So, when I asked him to join me in the Livestrong program as my support person, he didn't hesitate. Neil also enjoyed our Taco Tuesdays and talking with the other men. Through every exercise session, he sported a smile on his sweet face.

As the final bell rang, marking the end of our twelve-week program, our tribe made a pact to never let go of each other. We vowed to meet every Tuesday for a sweat-drenched workout and a Taco Tuesday feast. The bond forged between us, once strangers but now friends, is unbreakable, and I know we will be connected for life.

Thank you to the YMCA for the Livestrong Program.

***

Internet Research:

Older women, breast cancer, and social support - PMC (nih.gov)

Social support is characterized as any combination of emotional, tangible, appraisal, and informational support. Support can be formal, informal, social, professional, structured, or unstructured . It has been recognized for many years that social support is an important factor which may affect the general well-being of individuals living with chronic and life-threatening health conditions like breast cancer . Social support can help women with breast cancer to adjust and cope, and can have positive impacts on the survivor's health For an individual who has completed treatment, social support can enhance her quality of life and ease her transition into life after treatment For breast cancer survivors, access to a supportive environment can prevent long-term psychological difficulties and benefit her general well-being.

***

Today's Quote:

"Plenty of people will think you're crazy, no matter what you do. Don't let that stop you from finding the people who think you're incredible - the ones who need to hear your voice because it reminds them of their own. Your tribe.

They're out there. Don't let your critics interfere with your search for them."

—Vironika Tugaleva

A Note to You:

My dear pink sister, the journey of breast cancer can be a lonely and frightening one, but finding your tribe is crucial. Don't be afraid to reach out for support through programs like Livestrong, in-person support groups, or online communities on platforms such as Facebook. And if you can't find a group that resonates with you, consider creating your own. It doesn't have to be anything elaborate - even meeting for coffee monthly can make a world of difference. Together, we are stronger, and we will get through this journey together.

Cancer Post #91: No More: November 25th

Excruciating joint pain that caused me to cry out when trying to stand from my chair, along with my declining cognitive abilities, made me realize I couldn't take it anymore. As earlier mentioned, my oncologist and I decided to switch medications after a two-week break from Letrozole.

During the initial two weeks of being off the medication, I experienced a significant improvement in my overall well-being. I felt like a million bucks! My energy levels improved, and I felt terrific. My friends and family kept commenting on how much better I looked and how the old Shelley was back.

The nurse assured me she would call at the end of my two weeks, but the weeks passed without any communication. As I prepared to start the new medication, the lack of interaction made me question my decision. I saw the no-call as a sign not to experiment with a different brand of hormone blocker.

After praying intently, I made the decision to forego trying a different brand of blockers. Despite this choice, I couldn't shake the gut feeling that I would never be at peace with any medical decisions regarding my cancer if they went against my doctor's orders. Many oncologists pressure survivors to continue taking these medications because they believe in the percentages of the med's effectiveness. But do they truly understand the toll it takes?

If I were younger or in a more advanced stage of cancer, I might have been willing to endure the side effects. But at this point in my life, I value the next five years as potentially my last ones without the pains of aging. I've decided to prioritize quality of life over quantity and am fully aware of the consequences. Of course, I hope luck is on my side, and I never experience a recurrence of cancer. I also pray for advancements in treatments and cures that are less harsh on the body.

My mind whirled with conflicting thoughts as I came to terms with my decision to stop taking the drug. However, a sense of calm washed over me when I thought about the end of my life. Despite any regrets or mistakes, I've lived a rich and full life filled with extraordinary days and remarkable people for whom I'm grateful. And yet, there are things I have done that weigh heavy on my heart, and things I have yet to do that must be done. Whether time is on my side or not, I'm determined to cherish each day as if it were a precious gift, embracing every moment and opportunity that comes my way.

Determined to lower my estrogen levels without medication, I politely declined the decadent homemade desserts that were offered to me. Sugar creates weight gain, which produces fat, which creates estrogen. I explained to the person who made the sweet treat, I would love to eat it, but I was focused on using nutrition as a form of healing. I also committed to increasing my physical activity. Knowing my tendency towards perfectionism, I consciously tried to forgive myself when I slipped up and not give up on my plan altogether. Gradually, I learned to be more forgiving and gentler with myself on this journey towards better health.

I pulled my dad's letter out of my memory box, written several years before he died. On one hand, his words of not wanting to be mourned made sense - why would he want us to cry for him? But on the other hand, it was hard to just remember the good times and ignore the pain of losing him. My cancer helped me finally understand what he was saying. Here is his quote from the letter. "Don't cry for me when I am gone. Remember the good times. Remember how much I loved you."

***

Internet Research:

15 Cancer Fighting Foods (veryhealthy.life)

It is probably fair to say that food alone cannot contain or cure your cancer – but nutrition has a big role to play along with other remedies – conventional or not – in giving your body the best shot at healing itself.

***

Today's Quote:

"Do not reward yourself with food. You are not a dog."

—Unknown

A Note to You:

Breast cancer is a never-ending battlefield, filled with difficult decisions and constant uncertainty. It's like walking on a tightrope made of flames, stretching into an endless abyss. We all wish for a crystal ball to guide us through the smoke and chaos, but the reality is that every choice we make feels like a gamble. And even when we finally decide, it can feel like building a house of cards, fragile and easily shattered. But my dear friend, try to find peace in your choices. I know it's easier said than done. Hugs to you as you navigate this journey.

SHELLEY MALICOTE STUTCHMAN

NOTES AND THOUGHTS

Chapter Thirty

TWENTY THOUSAND DOLLAR BOOBS

Cancer Post #92: Reconstruction: November 28th

After enduring numerous surgeries, I triumphantly arrived at the climax - breast reconstruction. The bill totaled a staggering $20,000, but thankfully, my insurance came through. Who would have thought each breast would carry a price tag of $10,000? Guess I'll have to start cherishing the girls like priceless gems.

I wanted to be open about my reconstruction if other women were interested in asking about it. But I drew the line at flashing.

A few days before my scheduled surgery, I woke up in the middle of the night with flu symptoms. I left a voicemail for my doctor, hoping the surgery could still go as planned.

As the thought of going under anesthesia once again crossed my mind, a wave of apprehension washed over me. The memories of my previous surgeries flooded back, each one accompanied by a lingering sense of unease. A friend had recently shared with me the tragic story of a woman who had undergone multiple cancer surgeries and treatments, only to meet her untimely demise on the operating table during her reconstruction. It was later discovered that the doctor had failed to check her labs before proceeding with the surgery, and her already weakened body could not handle the added trauma. I felt a sense of weariness when she told me the story of her friend. Word of advice: don't share stories like my friend did with me about someone dying when they're facing the same type of surgery.

***

Internet Research:

https://goaskalice.columbia.edu/

Now that the leak has been discovered, what's the risk to your health? There are a lot of misconceptions out there about ruptures, including people who say that a rupture can lead to tissue disease, breast cancer, or reproductive diseases. Rest assured, though: the FDA has found no evidence that any of these health conditions are associated with leaking implants.

***

Today's Quote:

"Through strength, I will mend."

—Anonymous

A Note to You:

I can feel your excitement bubbling up as you get closer to your reconstruction! Just imagine how confident and fabulous you'll look in your favorite outfits. And hey, some women choose not to have reconstruction at all and rock their flat chests with pride. They've had their fill of surgeries, and it's time to celebrate. So, let's raise a glass and say hip, hip, hooray for us!

Cancer Post #93: Random Thoughts: November 29th

The day before my reconstructive surgery, you could describe my mood in one word: grumpy. Even though I wanted this surgery, I dreaded the recovery process. Silly thoughts ran through my head like, what if my new breasts looked too perky or too large and made me resemble a sixty-seven-year-old porn star?

***

Internet Research:

What Are Intrusive Thoughts? And How To Stop Them (clevelandclinic.org)

"Sometimes, thoughts can be just completely random, and you go, "Wow, where did that come from?" says Dr. Alexander. "But a lot of times, intrusive thoughts are related to something that you're already anxious about."

***

Today's Quote:

"Try calling someone just to tell them you can't talk right now."

—Anonymous

A Note to You:

Random thoughts can be a strange and sometimes humorous part of the cancer journey. Like the one I had about looking like a retired porn star. But not all thoughts are light-hearted. Some can be unsettling and cause anxiety. If you can't shake these thoughts, it may be helpful to talk to a therapist. It's important to address any underlying anxieties during this challenging time. Trust me, as a fellow survivor, I know there is much to be anxious about on this journey.

Cancer Post #94: The Last Incision: November 30th

I shuffled through the mundane tasks of checking in for surgery and signing forms left and right. My anxiety built with each pen stroke, but my fears were eased when I met the anesthesiologist. His round face, rosy cheeks, and a joyful twinkle in his eyes reminded me of Santa Claus. He asked about my recent bout of respiratory flu and examined my throat with a tiny flashlight. After his thorough assessment, he declared me fit for surgery with a jovial pat on the back. I half expected to hear a Ho Ho Ho come out of him as he explained the anesthesia process and assured me of constant monitoring. His twinkling eyes and warm demeanor filled me with confidence. I knew I was in good hands with this skilled anesthesiologist who looked like St. Nick.

The surgery took two and a half hours. I couldn't wait to see my new breasts, but I knew I had to be patient until my follow-up appointment when the doctor would unwrap them. However, the doctor warned us they wouldn't be perfectly symmetrical for a while, if ever. My husband replied, "I don't care about perfect breasts. I care about Shelley."

***

Internet Research:

After breast reconstruction: what to expect | Breast Cancer Now

Adjusting to how your reconstructed breast looks and feels can take time. It can take several months for your reconstructed breast to heal and settle and for your scars to fade. It's important you're satisfied with the final look and feel. If you're unhappy with the size or shape of the reconstructed breast or your other breast, let your breast care nurse or surgeon know. They can talk to you about possible options.

PEEK-A-BOOB

***

Today's Quote:

"If he only wants you for your breasts, legs, and thighs, send him to KFC."

—Drake

A Note to You:

I know it's tempting to sneak a peek at your new body after surgery, but believe me, following the doctor's orders will give you the best results. You've already come so far in this journey. Don't jeopardize your progress by rushing things. Trust the process and take care of yourself.

Cancer Post #95: Perky: December 1st

I awoke to my first post-operative day with the sun shining through the window. A wave of optimism washed over me. I felt perky. I took in the sweet aroma of freshly brewed coffee, brought to me by my loving husband while I was still nestled under the covers. Those small and thoughtful gestures hold such significance in my heart.

After my coffee I checked into my patient portal. I read the online report. I had no idea what it meant so I researched with Dr. Google. The one thing I knew, I was sure glad to see those last three words, negative for malignancy. The report read: In formalin labeled "Stutchman, Shelley, left breast anterior capsule" is fibrotic capsular fragments with attached fat, 4.5 x 3.2 x 1.9 cm aggregate. Sectioned entirely A1-A2. Negative for malignancy.

***

Internet Research:

Capsular fibrosis with breast implants - The Aesthetics Dr. Rolf Bartsch & Dr. Katrin Batsch Plastic Surgery & Aesthetic Medicine

It is important to know that capsular fibrosis is not dangerous per se. It is not an infection, but in many cases only an aesthetic problem. However, severe capsular fibrosis can cause pain because the fiber bundles pull on the surrounding tissue. Capsular fibrosis often occurs after radiotherapy for breast tumors.

***

Today's Quote:

"When life kicks you, let it kick you forward."

—Kay Yow

A Note to You:

Once the final surgery is behind you, a weight is lifted. The world just seems brighter, and laughter comes easier. And suddenly, every day feels like a hug. But what I didn't expect was this overwhelming desire to help other women on their own pink journey. We all need a sister by our side through it all.

Cancer Post #96: The Heavy Burden: December 2nd

Imagine my surprise! I underwent surgery on Wednesday, and as a result, my appetite was suppressed. Come Friday, I was eager to see how much weight I had lost. But when I stepped on the scale…what? It showed that I had gained eight pounds instead! How could that be?

***

Internet Research:

Unforeseen Reasons For Weight Gain After Surgery - Health Guide Net

Weight gain immediately after surgery is a common finding. Fluid retention is actually a normal reaction to surgery due to the fact that the body releases ADH, a type of hormone that makes you hold onto fluid. Fluid retention typically lasts for about 5 days, then stops.

***

Today's Quote:

"I'm not gaining weight; I'm retaining awesomeness."

—Unknown

A Note to You:

Cancer is always full of tricks. After my surgery, I had no idea that I would suddenly gain so much water weight! I almost fainted when I saw the numbers on the scale. Don't be afraid to share strange side effects or emotions with fellow warriors. Knowing we're not alone in this rollercoaster ride is a relief.

Cancer Post #97: Peak-A-Boob: December 3rd

I finally got to take my first post-op shower. I unwound the dressings and took off the corset, and what to my wandering eyes should appear? Two perfect bumps on my chest, and I let out a cheer. The bumps looked so lively and fine I gave a wink and knew in a moment everything was in sync.

As I stood in front of the full-length mirror, I smiled at the success of my battle against cancer. My breasts bore the scars of multiple surgeries, but I wore them as badges of honor. The skilled surgeon left me with two perfect boobs, in my opinion. It was clear I had come full circle - both in my battle against cancer and in accepting my imperfections as a part of who I am. I remembered how my body and fashion choices had evolved over the decades, and different scars from different eras held memories.

In junior high, my sole mission was to achieve cuteness—not just any kind of cute, but the coveted cheerleader cute. I spent hours scouring fashion magazines and studying the popular girls in school, determined to emulate their shiny, long hair and chic outfits. Despite my efforts, I never made the cheerleading squad. But my parents were always there to support me, making sure I had the latest trends. My dad always beamed with pride at how adorable he thought I looked.

During my high school years, my main goal was to look hot and draw attention. The popular fashion at the time included halter tops, which always made my dad cringe when I left the house with a makeshift bandana shirt.

When motherhood descended upon me, I felt a newfound desire to present myself as put together and polished. I wanted to set an example for my children to show them the importance of good grooming. Standing in front of the mirror each morning, I carefully selected and arranged my clothes, making sure every wrinkle was smoothed and every button properly fastened. I took extra care with my hair and makeup, wanting to exude confidence and grace. As I walked out the door, I carried myself with poise, knowing that my appearance was not just a reflection of myself but also the values I hoped to instill in my children.

When I re-entered the workforce, I aimed to strike the perfect balance between attractiveness and professionalism. Most days, I settled on a fitted blazer over a silk blouse paired with form-fitting trousers or a pencil skirt and sleek heels.

Surviving cancer opened a new chapter in my life, but I felt torn about how to present myself. On the one hand, I wanted to exude elegance and grace, a symbol of triumph over such a difficult battle. On the other hand, cancer taught me to appreciate and honor my body for its resilience. When I looked in the mirror, I struggled between who was I now, and how did I want the world to see me?

***

Internet Research:

Breast Augmentation Recovery Process and Timeline (healthline.com)

Breast augmentation recovery usually takes 6 to 8 weeks. It might be longer if you develop complications, like an infection or implant leak.

To ensure a smooth recovery, follow your surgeon's instructions. Wear the recovery bra, and care for your incision sites as directed. Be sure to get plenty of rest and eat a healthy diet. You should be fully recovered and ready to resume normal activities in about eight weeks.

***

Today's Quote:

"I believe one can live many lives through personal style. Every day is an occasion to reinvent yourself."

—Ralph Lauren

A Note to You:

We need every woman to see us survivors as symbols of strength and resilience, a living testament showing we can conquer this merciless disease that ravages our bodies and shatters our self-worth. We are a tribe of warriors, picking ourselves up from the wreckage of surgeries, treatments, and medications and bravely beginning anew. That is why I embrace elegance in this next chapter of my life. Because we, the sisterhood of breast cancer survivors, epitomize grace and beauty in the face of adversity.

However, when Christmas comes, I will proudly don my horrendously tacky Christmas sweaters, but fear not, for I shall do so with utmost style and grace.

Cancer Post #98: Perseverance's Promise: December 5th

When I reached this pivotal point in the story, I realized there was still so much more to tell. As you have journeyed through the pages of this book, you've witnessed how my emotions ran deep and wild. From spiritual battles and anger mixed with gratitude towards the medical system to moments of wanting to give up, my story has been a rollercoaster of feelings. But in the midst of it all, something shifted. I began to see the silver linings, the blessings cancer brought into my life. New friendships formed, a newfound appreciation for each day and all its little wonders, a deeper capacity for love, a determination to check items off of my bucket list, and a commitment to take care of my body. Most importantly, I learned to let go of things that were causing me stress and focus on what truly matters in life. Through cancer, I found peace and clarity amidst the chaos.

I went back to my hometown for a late Thanksgiving celebration. I sat on the couch in my daughter's living room, surrounded by the warmth and laughter of my family. My two grandsons were sprawled out on the floor, along with my four energetic great-grandchildren. As I watched them, a realization hit me like a warm wave - I will never truly disappear. A piece of me will always live on in each of these precious babies, and even as they grow up and have children of their own, that connection to me will remain. It was a humbling and beautiful revelation, and I closed my eyes for a moment to silently thank all of my ancestors who came before me who led me to this moment in my life.

Despite my physical limitations from the recent reconstruction surgery, my family took great care to ensure I didn't strain myself. My grandson's girlfriend, now his wife, graciously poured my iced tea so I wouldn't have to lift the heavy jug. My grandson attended to my every need with unwavering devotion. I got to meet my new precious great-grandson for the first time, though I couldn't hold him in my arms. His toothless grin filled me with joy and reminded me that life continues to bring blessings. Life moves forward.

***

Internet Research:

Does DNA Get Washed Out Over Generations? - Who are You Made Of?

How many generations back does DNA go?

There is no hard and fast answer that applies to everyone, but there are a few things that we do know for sure. For example, we will always inherit substantial percentages of DNA from:

• parents (50%)

• grandparents (about 25%)

• great-grandparents (about 12.5%)

• great-great-grandparents (about 6.25%)

• great-great-great grandparents (about 3.125%)

***

Today's Quote:

"Genetic code is a divine writing."

—Toba Beta

A Note to You:

It warms my heart to think that a piece of me will continue through the generations. My dear friend, take a moment to smile and bask in the beauty of those little ones in your family. Have you ever considered jotting down your unique traits and passing those pieces of information along to your loved ones? It's like spreading love and sunshine for years to come. They'll know where their love of music or sports ability, or whatever it is that makes you who you are, came from, and carry a piece of you with them always.

Cancer Post #99: Squeak: December 8th

A good doctor should have a sense of humor. At my follow-up appointment with my plastic surgeon, I decided to have a little fun. I brought along a squeaky dog toy and concealed it in my hand. When the surgeon reached out to touch my breast, I squeezed the toy, and she let out a scream, jumping back in surprise. I couldn't resist asking, "Did you put a squeaker in there during the surgery?"

Her laughter was loud and genuine, filling the room with a symphony of joy and amusement.

After our sides had stopped aching from the fit of laughter, the mood shifted back to solemnity. I told the doctor I was worried because I was tired. My surgeon's expression turned sympathetic as she reminded me of all the factors at play—a recent virus, three surgeries in just five months, and not being a young spring chicken anymore. She reassured me time would be my ally in regaining my strength and vitality.

My doctor then said, "We found a small mass in your left breast during the reconstruction surgery." My heart dropped. "But don't worry," she added quickly, "we tested it, and it's benign."

Despite her reassurance, anxiety gnawed at me. Ever since my cancer diagnosis, every abnormality felt like a looming threat. I needed to remind myself not to jump to conclusions and trust the doctor's expertise.

I was cleared to return to work on Dec. 20th but with a weight restriction of only lifting something five pounds or less. My doctor reminded me I was still healing and shouldn't push myself too hard. Also, my exercise was limited to walking only. She would recheck me on Jan. 19th and hopefully loosen the restrictions.

I will never forget when I left the building that day, I said a little prayer that I was coming to the end of this journey and would see less of hospitals and doctors in the New Year.

***

Internet Research:

https://thewonderlist.net/doctor-humour-15-health-specialist-who-know-how-to-have-a-laugh

Luckily doctors have a good sense of humor, as their daily workload is not always a bundle of laughs. Between tragic outcomes to deliver to close relatives, the fear of being unable to save someone's life, and the stress of the operating table where you need to be constantly on high alert, a bit of humor and carefree banter never goes a miss.

***

Today's Quote:

"I saw a woman wearing a sweatshirt with 'Guess' on it...

So, I said, 'Implants?'"

—Author Unknown

A Note to You:

It takes serious guts to prank your doctor. However, if you muster up the courage it is well worth the laughter. I wish for you every day is filled with a spark in your eye and a contagious giggle that fills the air. Be a little mischievous, pink sister.

Cancer Post #100: Bras: December 18th

My obsession with breast cancer consumed me, driving me to devour every piece of information I found. As I delved deeper into my research, one study stated - wearing a bra can actually cause cancer. The very undergarment that society deems necessary for women was now a potential threat to their lives. But in a sick twist of fate, I found myself secretly thrilled by this discovery. I hated wearing bras.

Throughout my extensive research on breast cancer, I've come to realize the importance of not relying on a single source. The abundance of information available makes it difficult to distinguish fact from fiction. While putting my trust in doctors may seem logical, I've noticed a trend of similar treatment protocols being prescribed for all patients, which raises concerns about individual needs and circumstances being overlooked. It's clear we still have much to learn about cancer, as evidenced by the lack of a cure. I hope this is due to the complexity of the disease rather than financial motives within the medical industry.

As I delved deeper into the ongoing debate about whether women should wear bras or not, I began to lean towards the conclusion that wearing or not wearing a bra had no correlation with an increased risk of developing breast cancer. It's frustrating not to have a reliable way to differentiate between fact and fiction. If only I had a crystal ball.

***

Internet Research:

Do Bras Cause Breast Cancer? - Ask Dr. Weil (drweil.com)

According to the American Cancer Society (ACS), the idea that bras can cause breast cancer comes from a book published in the 1990s called Dressed to Kill by a husband-and-wife team of medical anthropologists who suggested that bras compress the breasts' lymphatic system, resulting in an accumulation of cancer-causing toxins. The ACS notes on its website that the study purporting to establish this link "was not conducted according to standard principles of epidemiological research" and did not take into consideration other variables, including the known risks for breast cancer. What's more, the idea that bras lead to blocked lymphatic vessels and accumulation of toxins "is inconsistent with scientific concepts of breast physiology and pathology," the ACS explains.

***

Today's Quote:

"Bras are often booby-trapped."

—Tiffany Reisz

A Note to You:

Bras the ever-present necessary evil in a woman's wardrobe. They can make us feel sexy or suffocated, depending on the day. Who came up with the brilliant idea to strap our girls into these contraptions? It's like forcing men to wear neckties but for our boobs. Why can't we just go around braless and free like men do with their nipples? #freethenipple

NOTES AND THOUGHTS

CHAPTER THIRTY-ONE

MY HALLMARK CHRISTMAS

Cancer Post #101: Christmas: December 26th

I absolutely adore Hallmark Christmas movies! From the day after Thanksgiving until Christmas Day, I indulge in one after the other. Even though I understand these movies are purely fictional and depict a world that's too perfect, I secretly hoped to have my own Hallmark picture-perfect Christmas someday.

My Hallmark Christmas happened the year of my breast cancer.

Let me paint the picture for you. My husband and I, newlyweds of only six months, worked together through three cancer surgeries. As a result, my energy levels were almost non-existent, and I felt like a burden to him at times. My reconstruction surgery was on November 30th, and my doctor had instructed me to rest as much as possible and not exert myself. With it being the holiday season, I decided to use this time to recover by snuggling under a warm blanket on the couch and binge-watching Christmas movies from Hallmark. Since my hearing has declined, possibly due to age, I would have the TV turned up loud and wouldn't even hear my husband enter the living room until he started grumbling about my movie choices. "How can you watch so many Hallmark Christmas movies?" he would mutter in frustration.

His words were a mixture of curiosity and skepticism as he spoke. I could never quite tell if it was a question or a statement that lingered on his tongue. "They all have the same plot," he would muse.

A grin spread across my face as I responded, "That's one of the movie's most endearing qualities."

On the Wednesday before Christmas day, I met my husband and his friend Bill for a drink at a local bar. As we sipped our drinks, we chatted about our impending holiday plans. I explained the significance of waking up on Christmas morning to find something special in my stocking.

The guys were all ears, or just being polite, as I shared my tale. As a child in school, I would hear my classmates chatting about the goodies they found in their Christmas stockings. I asked my mother why I never received one, and she would always reply, "That isn't a part of our family tradition."

As a child, simple explanations did nothing to quell my desire for a stocking. So, the following year, I hatched a plan. I carefully selected one of my favorite socks. I hung it in a prominent spot in the house, where Santa and my parents could easily spot it. I eagerly raced to my stocking on Christmas morning, anticipation bubbling inside me.

But alas, it was empty. Don't get me wrong, my parents were wonderful and loving and showered me with gifts. Christmas Stockings just didn't seem important to them.

Despite my disappointment from the previous year, I couldn't resist hanging my stocking again for Christmas. This time, I devised an even better plan than before. Whenever someone gave me a penny, I stuffed it into my stocking, hoping my parents and Santa would catch on and fill it with goodies. When I woke up on Christmas morning, I dashed to my stocking with eager anticipation. But to my chagrin, there were only the pennies I put in. Though disappointed, I lifted my spirits by counting all the change. The total added up to enough for me to buy a candy bar and an ice-cold Coke from the gas station. I never dared to hang a stocking again.

Flash forward to the present. That is how the movies do it, isn't it?

I hung the Christmas stockings that Melissa, Neil's daughter, had lovingly made for our wedding. I checked my stocking every day, only to find it empty. I couldn't help feeling a twinge of disappointment. I knew I should let it go and focus on the joyous holiday season ahead.

On Christmas morning, my stocking overflowed with treats: a gift card to Sonic, a spa day voucher, and other small presents. But my heart skipped a beat when I reached into the depths of the sock and felt something heavy inside a tiny baggie. I pulled out the bag, revealing a handful of shiny pennies that glinted in the light like precious jewels. Tears welled in my eyes as I realized the sentimental value behind my husband's simple yet meaningful gesture.

I got my Hallmark Christmas movie moment.

***

Internet Research:

Hallmark (komen.org)

Since 1999, Hallmark designs a new limited edition Hallmark Keepsake Ornament to benefit Komen. Hallmark customers view Hallmark Keepsake Ornaments as more than just a holiday decoration. Each year as customers place their ornaments on their trees, it helps them relive special memories and show support for the breast cancer community.

***

Today's Quote:

"Dammit I fell asleep during a Hallmark movie so now I'll never know if the cute couple who misunderstood each other at first fell in love."

—Kim Bongiorno

A Note to You:

Girlfriend, if you're as obsessed with Hallmark movies as I am, I'm sending you all the warm and fuzzy vibes for a perfect Hallmark moment in your own life. Don't forget our loved ones can't always read our minds, so don't be afraid to tell them what you need during this tough holiday season while battling cancer. Don't hesitate to create your own special moments. Treat yourself to some pink flowers, a cozy candle, and delicious sugar cookies, and indulge in a marathon of your favorite feel-good movies. Sending all my love to my fellow pink sisters.

…

NOTES AND THOUGHTS

CHAPTER THIRTY-TWO

THE WHY'S

Cancer Post #102: I Got Cancer Because: December 28th

My dear friend Claudette surprised me with Chris Wark's ultimate DVD set. This revolutionary program delves into the power of food, prayer, exercise, rest, forgiveness, and stress management in healing cancer. As I eagerly dove into the first disc, Chris's question echoed in my mind: "Why do you believe you have cancer?"

That is a serious question. I rolled it over and over in my mind, but never took the time to get a piece of paper and pencil and write down my thoughts on this fundamental question. Those answers stared back at me when I penned my thoughts on paper. I wish I had paid better attention to my health. I hope when you read my list if you notice something you may be doing that increases your chances of getting cancer or a recurrence, you will be motivated to take corrective action before some doctor calls you and says those dreaded words, "Your cancer is back."

HRT:
I took hormone replacement therapy from when I turned fifty-seven until the day I received my diagnosis at age sixty-seven. I knew that I was playing with fire by taking HRT because my mother and sister both had breast cancer. So, you may wonder, "Why did I do it?"

The doctors' claims were my shield as I blindly trusted in their assurances. They preyed on my fear of aging, promising youth and vitality through hormone replacement therapy. My ego was stroked with talk of staying slim, maintaining a full head of hair, and having strong bones and skin that defied the march of time. And let's not forget about my sexual desires - they would be at peak levels thanks to HRT. The words " small risk of b reast cancer" were overshadowed by the alluring benefits promised by these doctors who were interested in fattening their wallets with my hard-earned money. How could I resist such seductive promises?

It's worth repeating: the doctors assured me that HRT had a very low risk of breast cancer. They capitalized on our societal belief that we are at our prime in our twenties when our hormones are raging. Their persuasive language appealed to my vanity, and I rationalized that the potential benefits outweighed the slight chance of developing breast cancer.

I must confess, hormone replacement therapy did seem to do what the doctors claimed. But not one of those doctors warned me that consistently adding estrogen to my body would heighten my chances of developing estrogen-positive cancer.

For those suffering from menopausal symptoms, Hormone Replacement Therapy (HRT) can be a godsend. The daily struggles and discomforts are alleviated, and we feel like ourselves again for a time. However, as with all things in life, there comes a time when we must face the consequences of our choices. Now that I have stopped my HRT regimen, I am facing severe hot flashes and the multitude of other physical and emotional challenges that come with menopause. Mother Nature may be fooled for a while. But eventually, she will catch up with us, reminding us of the natural cycle of life.

I couldn't help but think back to when I made the decision to start hormone replacement therapy. It seemed like a harmless choice at the time - what's a little extra estrogen to ward off wrinkles? But now, having faced the harsh reality of breast cancer, I wish I had dug deeper into the research and listened to my gut instinct. Was vanity worth risking my health? In hindsight, I would have gladly traded a few wrinkles for a healthier body and peace of mind.

Overweight:

At the age of fourteen, my struggle with weight commenced. It was a pivotal moment when my mother, a slender woman, took me to the doctor. Concerned about my weight gain, she hoped the doctor would provide some answers. And he did - I was overeating. From that day on, my battle with weight and body image began in earnest. I would sneak food and binge at night when my mother wasn't looking, followed by two days of fasting and only drinking water. Looking back, I now realize this was a form of disordered eating. It kept me slim and made my mother happy, but it also allowed me to indulge in all the food I wanted during my binges. One memory that will always stick with me is fainting during high school because I was on day three of a water fast. But even then, I couldn't bring myself to tell the nurse the real reason behind it.

When I reached adulthood, my body changed. Twenty-five pounds crept onto my frame. Frustrated and unhappy with my newfound weight, I turned to Weight Watchers to shed the extra pounds. It became a familiar cycle – gain, lose, repeat – one I would duplicate numerous times in the years to come.

As I came to terms with my diagnosis of estrogen-fed cancer, I couldn't help but regret my past choices. My constant indulgence in food and disregard for my health caught up with me, magnifying the production of estrogen in my body. I wish I had educated myself on proper nutrition and cared for my body instead of playing a dangerous game with food. The extra weight I carried may have played a role in developing breast cancer.

I also wish there was a magic pill that could cure my addiction to food. But every time I start eating healthier and making good choices, I eventually fall off the wagon and end up bingeing on junk food. It's a constant battle that feels like riding a never-ending struggle bus.

Now, every time I bring food to my lips, I ask myself, "Shelley, will this be the food that fuels another cancerous growth, or will it be the nourishment that protects me?"

I understand everything we consume can bring us closer to salvation or destruction. I encourage you to take control of your weight and eating habits to give your body a fighting chance against the dreaded C.

Stress:

We are repeatedly told that stress can lead to illness, with cancer being included on that list.

I know I have unnecessary stress I create myself. I schedule too many things, promise to do things for others, and worry I can't keep those promises. I stress about my grown children, my grandchildren, and my great-grandchildren.

They have financial, relationship, parenting, health, and job struggles. It pains me that I am unable to simply make their struggles disappear, especially when they may need financial assistance. However, with my limited resources as I near retirement, I must carefully budget and save for the future.

I stress about the stock market. Will I live long enough to recoup my losses?

I'm anxious when I suspect I have hurt someone's emotions. Most people may not think much of it, but I worry that my words or actions may have been inappropriate.

I stress that cancer might come back.

Whenever my memory fails me, I feel a surge of panic that may be the early signs of dementia. The thought of losing my ability to recall even the simplest details worries me.

I'm aware I should surrender my worries to the Lord. Occasionally, this approach helps for a short period, but then the worrying creeps back in compounding my stress because I am not faithful enough to let go of my concerns. It's a never-ending cycle.

Could my constant worrying and high-stress lifestyle have been another contributor to my diagnosis? I couldn't deny the possibility. Losing weight was one thing, but changing my mindset seemed almost impossible. I pondered more on Chris Wark's probing question: what had I done to create an environment in my body for cancer to thrive? Despite my discomfort, I continued to answer his questions honestly, knowing that if I wanted to heal, I would need to make some significant changes.

I know that finding true peace may be my most challenging task, but I am determined to conquer it to remain cancer-free. Whether through prayer and unbreakable faith or any means necessary, I will learn to let go of stress before it consumes me from within.

Sleep:

I used to believe cramming my days with as many amazing experiences as possible was the key to a fulfilling life. I saw sleep as an inconvenience, something I could easily sacrifice for more time awake. But now, after going through cancer, I realize the true importance of sleep. It's not just about feeling rested, but it's when our bodies repair and heal. Was my neglect of sleep a factor in developing cancer? Nowadays, I prioritize getting seven to eight hours of sleep and a bonus Sunday afternoon nap. The value of rest has become clear to me, even if it took a health scare to fully understand.

Please prioritize your sleep. Evaluate your current habits and make any necessary changes for your health.

Forgiveness:

It is easy for me to forgive others, but I struggle with showing myself the same kindness. Reflecting on my past mistakes and their impact on others can be difficult. This lack of self-forgiveness may have contributed to the development of my cancer, much like how stress can play a role. I need to let go of the past and focus on learning from my mistakes, using each day as an opportunity to improve. While this exercise of pinpointing potential reasons for my cancer is challenging, it allows me to confront any negative habits or behaviors that could potentially lead to illness. I encourage anyone, regardless of whether they have cancer or not, to reflect on their own actions and think about what changes they can make to promote better health.

Fake Butter:

I have consumed tons of fake butter to save calories. My vanity was at play again. I didn't just spray the butter on, I poured it on. I thought it was God's gift to dieters. I loved the taste.

My husband expressed concern about the Parkay 0-calorie spray I used and researched its ingredients. His findings made me reconsider the many diet products I consumed. To prioritize clean eating and minimize potential risks, I cut out zero-calorie products that may contain harmful chemicals.

After we studied the ingredients of the 0-calorie Parkay, I thought about all the products I used in my daily routine. The suntan lotions that promised a golden glow, the anti-aging creams that claimed to turn back time, and the deodorants that kept me fresh and dry. Could toxins be seeping through my skin and into my body from these products? I decided to opt for natural and chemical-free alternatives.

Wine:

Alcohol is also being scrutinized. I've managed to decrease my wine intake from eight glasses per week to only three drinks in the same time frame. It's still my guilty pleasure, as I haven't completely eliminated it.

In his book and videos, Chris Wark asked another hard question: "Do you really want to live?"

Wow, that was powerful. I had to think for a minute. Do I want to live bad enough that I will be committed to healthier living? A battle between instant gratification and long-term well-being waged within, each side vying for control. I chose to live.

***

Internet Research:

How I Used The Raw Vegan Diet to Beat Cancer Naturally (chrisbeatcancer.com)

The best source of clean, high-quality fuel for your body comes from raw organic fruits, vegetables, seeds, and nuts. This is food designed by God for us, His creation, to eat. But we've gotten away from that. Thanks to technological innovations and modern conveniences, the majority of the food we now eat in America is "processed." It is not natural, and it is not healthy. Processed food is junk food. Most of us think of junk food as soft drinks, candy, snacks, fast food, and tv dinners. But in reality, junk food is almost any food that has been altered by man and packaged for resale.

If you want to learn more about nutrition and cancer, check out Chris's website.

***

Today's Quote:

"If man made it, don't eat it."

—Jack LaLanne

A Note to You:

I know you've probably asked yourself a million times why this cancer crap happened to you. But instead of getting lost in the "whys," let's focus on the important questions - what are the whys running around in your head, and are you willing to keep fighting for your life? It won't be easy, but facing these tough realities will ultimately bring about change and make you even stronger.

Cancer Post #103: The Gastric Gambit: January 2nd

A nasty stomach bug took hold of me, forcing me to constantly sprint to the bathroom. It was not the way I wanted to kick off the New Year.

Being diagnosed with cancer changes everything. It's no longer just a stomach virus but a burden on my mind. Lying in bed, bundled under layers of blankets, my thoughts turned dark, and doubts crept in: could this be more than just a simple virus?

As my stomach churned, I thought - stomach cancer. But then my mind spiraled into a frenzy, considering every possible illness - colon cancer, liver disease, even pancreatic cancer. I tried calming myself down, reminding myself it was a simple stomach virus. But the fear didn't dissipate. Every little ache or pain made me worry about my health, and I wondered if I was turning into a hypochondriac.

I reached out to my Breast Cancer Facebook group, P31, and asked, "Am I nuts?"
As I read the other women's answers, my nerves calmed. Each woman shared stories of their own battles with cancer, recounting the constant anxiety they feel at any hint of illness or abnormality in their bodies. They spoke of the fear of recurrence. One woman summed it up beautifully. She explained when you get cancer, you have been through a traumatic event, and lumps, bumps, coughs, twitches, and anything that is out of the ordinary health-wise becomes a trigger. I remember what she said every time I started to panic. I won the cancer battle, and I won't let PTSD steal my peace.

***

Internet Research:

Why Is Fear Such a Problem With Breast Cancer? (usnews.com)

Fear goes along with breast cancer at virtually every step of the process. From the fear of waiting for a diagnosis to the ongoing fear of recurrence that follows survivors long after they've completed treatment, the anxiety of what lies ahead at every turn is a very real thing.

"It wasn't until after I had experienced cancer that I realized that really, what this is, is sort of a trigger for post-traumatic stress disorder – like a war veteran might [feel] if he hears a car backfire and thinks it's a gunshot and it reminds him of the gunshots he heard when he was fighting in the war. Sometimes, our studies or scans can trigger this post-traumatic stress disorder," Liberman says. The unpredictability of the outcome is the issue, and it gets triggered by the knowledge that the scan could lead to bad news.

***

Today's Quote:

"If you woke up this morning with more health than illness, you are more fortunate than the million people on the planet who will not survive this week. If you can attend a religious meeting without fear of harassment, arrest, torture, or death, you are more blessed than three billion people in the world."

—Ted Zeff

A Note to You:

My sweet friend, cancer is a never-ending battle for our sanity. Our friends may not understand why we constantly fear every cough and pain, wondering if the cancer has spread to our lungs. But I know, and so do our fellow pink sisters. So, let's be kind to ourselves when we have moments of panic. Just the other day, I burned my thumb on the stove and instantly worried about my left side, where I had lymphedema during my battle with breast cancer. It's been almost two years since I've been declared cancer-free, and yet the fear still lingers. It does get easier over time, I promise you that. We will always have some level of stress about our health, but we are fighters and will overcome anything that comes our way. Together, we are stronger than any disease.

NOTES AND THOUGHTS

CHAPTER THIRTY-THREE

INSURANCE, MEDICARE, PAYMENTS...OH MY

Cancer Post #104: Policy of Fury: January 6th

I became a grouchy bear when dealing with insurance companies.

I can empathize with the stress and frustration of receiving a bill that demands immediate payment or a callback, especially when there's confusion about the charges. I found myself in this situation when I received a bill from a facility urging me to pay or call them immediately. According to the bill, I owed $2,400.00 for a test done in July despite already fulfilling all my insurance deductions and out-of-pocket expenses. Determined to find an explanation, I called my insurance company. The process was daunting - navigating through automated menus and being put on hold for hours - only to be told I reached the wrong department. But I persisted and eventually spoke to a representative. I blurted out, "Why hasn't this bill been paid yet?"

She explained they sent the facility several notices requesting my medical records. "They never responded," she added.

Frustrated and armed with mad, I called the facility after I expressed concern about my credit being impacted. The woman on the other end assured me my bill would not be sent to collections. I explained my insurance company informed me they never received any records from their facility. I gave her the fax number where the information should be sent. "Please take care of this immediately," I said sternly.

The woman promised the billing error would be taken care of promptly.

To confirm the details of the pending charges were communicated, my husband recommended I call daily to ensure they did what they said they would. He is a retired CPA and gives me good suggestions about handling billing situations.

On the second day of phone calls, a new voice greeted me. She sounded tired but professional. "I see the note about sending your information," she said, her fingers typing away on a keyboard in the background.

"Have they sent the records?" I asked.

She replied, "I don't know."

With a hint of annoyance, I said, "I'll call every day. I need reassurance that the records are in the hands of the insurance company."

After a pause, she said, "Let me give you a different phone number to call." I heard a drop of malice in her voice.

On day #3, I called the new number. Exasperated, I restated my predicament and inquired if they had finally sent the records. The woman on the line replied nonchalantly, "Oh, we sent those back in November."

I explained to the representative the insurance company didn't receive the documents and requested they again be sent. The representative acknowledged my request. Exasperated, I told her I would call daily until I received confirmation everyone had the information needed to process the billing.

I heard her roll her eyes.

After my fourth call, I crossed my fingers and hoped for the best. Thankfully, everything fell into place, and the insurance company approved the bill. I worry about those who are too ill to fight this battle or don't fully comprehend the situation and end up paying anyway.

Many patients resort to hiring a professional patient advocate or seeking assistance from a nurse navigator.

***

Internet Research:

Common Errors in Medical Billing and Coding, and How to Avoid Them (mticollege.edu)

Medical billers and coders are crucial to the healthcare industry. They keep doctors and nurses on track and organized by carefully documenting patient procedures and treatments. In addition, they submit bills to insurance companies, which then pay claims. When a medical biller or coder makes a mistake, it can delay the claims process, cause a loss of revenue, and/or affect a patient's care.

Here is an interesting fact:

Because of a rapidly aging U.S. population, healthcare jobs are in demand because as people age, they usually need more medical care. According to the Bureau of Labor Statistics, the employment rate for medical records and health information technicians (billers and coders) is growing much faster than the average for other occupations because people in these jobs are the ones who handle insurance and patient claims.

***

Today's Quote:

"For every minute you are angry, you lose sixty seconds of happiness."

—Ralph Waldo Emerson

A Note for You:

I cringe when I remember how harshly I spoke to those insurance representatives. They were just doing their job and didn't deserve my anger. It's so essential for us women to stay calm and professional in these situations, even when it's frustrating. But don't give up, girl! Persistence is key. Don't hesitate to call them every day until your issue is resolved. And if you need some extra support, ask a friend or family member to be on the call with you and speak up on your behalf. We've got this, sister. Keep pushing until the job is done.

Cancer Post #105: Exploring Medicare: January 8th

Despite still being employed, I decided to switch to Medicare and leave behind the insurance provided by my company. The catalyst for this change was the realization that I would need to pay $3,000.00 out-of-pocket before my insurance would cover all expenses. With numerous tests already planned due to my battle with cancer, it was clear that switching to Medicare with its $200.00 deductible was the most practical option. The weight of medical costs felt like a never-ending burden. The promise of a lighter financial strain with Medicare brought a sense of relief.

When I signed up for Medicare B, my representative casually mentioned my monthly payment could potentially be higher if I had a good financial year based on my tax returns. But I didn't think much of what she said and thanked her for the information. However, when I received the letter from Medicare revealing my actual monthly payment, it was shockingly high. Tears welled in my eyes, and I couldn't believe how much more I would have to pay each month. It was a hard lesson learned about not fully understanding the details of my healthcare coverage.

My husband put his CPA skills to work and uncovered a loophole. He poured over pages of complicated regulations and stumbled upon it - a clause that could significantly lower my cost if I had experienced a major life change. I dialed Social Security, navigating through endless automated prompts until I finally reached a human representative after an hour on hold. I listened to her every word as she explained the SSA 44 form I needed to complete.

I filled out the SSA 44 form. Check. I drove to the SS office. Check. It should only take thirty minutes; what could go wrong? Famous last words. I left work at 2 p.m., and hours later, I was still there, just dropping off some "simple" paperwork.

After two and a half hours, I left the Social Security office, hoping I had filled out all the paperwork correctly.

***

Internet Research:

https://www.healthline.com/health/medicare/medicare-part-b-cost

However, the amount of this premium can increase based on your income. People with a higher income typically pay what's known as an income-related monthly adjustment amount.

***

Today's Quote:

"Give me six hours to chop down a tree and I will spend the first four sharpening the axe."

—Abraham Lincoln

My Note to You:

I know insurance and medical stuff can be a headache. Digging into the nitty-gritty is vital before jumping ship or finalizing any scheduled procedures. Don't just skim over the fine print - read it thoroughly and make sure you understand everything. You don't want any surprises. My husband saved my butt when we switched providers because he did his research. It could have been a costly disaster if he didn't. So, take your time and stay informed before making any big moves. Better safe than sorry, right?

NOTES AND THOUGHTS

Chapter Thirty-Four

HEARTBREAK LINKED TO BREAST CANCER

Cancer Post #106: Sick Heart: January 9th

Writing this post was quite challenging and painful for me.

For a while, I thought I knew the real reason why I got cancer. My cancer diagnosis at one time felt like a punishment, a consequence for my own wrongdoings. I carried the weight of guilt, knowing that it was my actions that led to the disintegration of my first marriage.

When the divorce was finalized, I would lay in bed and feel a sharp, stabbing pain in my chest - not just imagined, but as real as any physical injury.

My thoughts may seem irrational, but the sharp pang in my chest would make me wonder if the guilt would manifest itself physically, perhaps even leading to the development of breast cancer. That thought ran through my mind many times.

Four years later, a lump appeared on my breast, and the doctor confirmed it was cancer. Was it karma or just a coincidence? I believed my past actions had come back to haunt me in the form of this deadly disease.

***

Internet Research:

https://consumer.healthday.com/cancer-information-5/mis-cancer-news-102/can-a-broken-heart-contribute-to-cancer-

"Broken heart syndrome" may harm more than just the heart, new research suggests.

While the extreme stress of losing a loved one has been linked to heart troubles in prior research, a new study found that one in six people with broken heart syndrome also had cancer. Even worse, they were less likely to survive their cancer five years after diagnosis.

"There seems to be a strong interplay between Takotsubo syndrome [broken heart syndrome] and malignancies," said study senior author Dr. Christian Templin. He's director of acute cardiac care at University Hospital Zurich in Switzerland.

The new study included just over 1,600 people with broken heart syndrome. The participants were recruited at 26 medical centers in nine different countries, including eight European countries and the United States.

Among those diagnosed with cancer, most were women (88%) and their average age was seventy.

The most common type of cancer was breast cancer. Other cancers affected areas including the digestive system, the respiratory tract, internal sex organs and the skin.

**

Today's Quote:

"Turn down the volume of your negative inner voice and create a nurturing inner voice to take its place. When you make a mistake, forgive yourself, learn from it, and move on instead of obsessing about it. Equally important, don't allow anyone else to dwell on your mistakes or shortcomings or to expect perfection from you."

—Beverly Engel

A Note to You:

I finally let go of all the self-blame and guilt. It took a lot of therapy and prayer, but I'm in a better place now. Of course, there are still moments when those feelings resurface, but I've learned to breathe deeply and practice positive self-talk. I found it interesting there's a link between a broken heart and breast cancer. It's crazy how much our emotional well-being can affect our physical health. By finally forgiving myself, I'm back in a good place. If you need to forgive yourself for anything, take a moment right now to do it. Whether through prayer or speaking it aloud to the universe, remind yourself that you are good, whole, and forgiven. Love to you, my pink sister.

NOTES AND THOUGHTS

Chapter Thirty-Five

I BOOKED A CRUISE AND OTHER RANDOM THINGS

Cancer Post #107: Seven Months: January 10th

January marked seven months of being cancer-free for me, a milestone I celebrated with joy. The number seven is often associated with good luck, so I took it as a positive sign to start the new year with my seven-month anniversary.

We celebrated the milestone by going to dinner with my Livestrong tribe. When I talked to the manager, I felt a surge of pride for the journey all the ladies sitting at the table went through. I proudly told the server, "It's my seven-month cancer-free anniversary."

With a hint of slyness, I may have subtly mentioned our survivor status in hopes of receiving a complimentary dessert. Sadly, my charm did not sway the waiter, but the evening still overflowed with laughter and love.

***

Internet Research:

10 ways to celebrate your cancerversary | Edward-Elmhurst Health (eehealth.org)

Getting through the different phases of the cancer journey is a big deal. Setting milestones can help you stay positive and motivated, and overcome hurdles along the way.

Whatever your milestones may be, when you reach one, be sure to acknowledge it. For instance, some people remember their "cancerversary" as the day they were told they were cancer-free or the day they finished treatment. Every cancerversary, they find a way to celebrate in a way that makes sense for them.

***

Today's Quote:

"My cancer scare changed my life. I'm grateful for every new, healthy day I have. It has helped me prioritize my life."

—Olivia Newton-John

A Note to You:

My dear friend, embrace every milestone and cherish each cancer-free month as a reminder of your strength and desire to live. Take off your shoes, feel the earth beneath your feet, and hug a tree in gratitude for life's beauty. And most importantly, remember to wrap your arms around the people you love and celebrate every moment together. You are a warrior, my friend, and I am honored to celebrate this life with you.

Cancer Post #108: Cruise: January 13th

Cancer makes you reflect a lot. I thought about all the things I still wanted to do in life. But then a sobering thought hit me - what if there wasn't enough time? So, in a moment of spontaneity, I opened my laptop and booked a cruise for myself, my two grown children, and my bonus children. My wasbund and husband never wanted to go on a cruise, but I dreamed of cruising. My kids and bonus kids were as excited about this experience as me. We would sail across the ocean together, making new memories and cherishing our ocean adventure.

The day after I impulsively booked the luxurious cruise, reality hit me hard when I received my W-2 from work. The significant drop in my income due to all the time off I had taken made me question if I could actually afford this trip. The thought of canceling the cruise crossed my mind, questioning if I should spend extra thousands on something I couldn't afford. Yet, I still held onto that desire for adventure and luxury. The internal battle between practicality and indulgence waged on in my mind.

The realization crashed over me like a tidal wave - my existence was not guaranteed for the next day, year, or decade. Cancer propelled me to form a bucket list, determined to make every moment count. I hoped our blended family would have each other's backs in my absence. I wanted them to forge a solid bond to withstand any tumult they may face together as one unit. I hoped the cruise would unite my kids and bonus kids as one.

The following morning, I opened my eyes and took a deep breath. Gratitude filled my heart. The sun shining through the blinds, the warmth of my bed, and the opportunity to go on a dream cruise. Cancer may have been a difficult obstacle, but it ultimately led me to take this leap and fulfill a long-held desire. Thank you, cancer, for pushing me towards this incredible experience.

I call my children "kids," even though they are all in their forties. Despite my worries about the money I wasn't earning and the declining stock market, I felt joy that we were embarking on an adventure together. I trusted that after the cruise, my concerns about a lower W-2 or shrinking investments would fade away, replaced by cherished memories. The decreased balance in my bank account wouldn't hold much weight compared to the priceless time spent with my adult children.

That day, I paid for the cruise in full. We were scheduled to set sail in April.

***

Internet Research:

Emotions and Cancer - NCI

Some people see their cancer as a "wake-up call." They realize the importance of enjoying the little things in life. They go places they've never been. They finish projects they had started but put aside. They spend more time with friends and family. They mend broken relationships.

***

Today's Quote:

"Jobs fill your pocket, but adventures fill your soul."

—Jamie Lyn Beatty

A Note to You:

Before cancer, my life was filled with a lot of 'what ifs.' I would weigh the benefits and consequences. I overthought almost every decision, which sometimes led to no decision. No decision would mean my life didn't move forward or backward; it flatlined. Let your cancer be a reminder to always pursue your dreams and take bold steps toward a brighter future. Let the adventures begin, my friend.

Cancer Post #109
Sunscreen Lotions:
January 18th

After being diagnosed with cancer, your awareness and caution towards the products you use increases. You start questioning whether they contain any ingredients that are known to cause cancer.

Because I would be using a lot of sunscreens on the family cruise, I researched suntan lotions. Houston, we have a problem.

***

Internet Research:

Cancer-Causing Chemicals in Sunscreens? Here's What You Need to Know | Resource | Baptist Health South Florida

Just as families across the U.S. look forward to spending more time outdoors this summer comes the unwelcome news that a number of popular sunscreens have been shown to contain benzene, a chemical known to cause leukemia and other blood cancers. Benzene is used primarily as a solvent in the chemical and pharmaceutical industries, and its use is tightly regulated.

Either way, says Dr. Kasper, benzene is not an ingredient that should be there, and consumers need to educate themselves on the different types of sunscreens available and the ingredients they contain.

Benzene contamination has not been found in any mineral-based sunscreens, and Dr. Kasper says these products are absolutely safe to use.

***

Today's Quote:

"Never bet with anyone you meet on the first tee who has a deep suntan, a 1-iron in his bag, and squinty eyes."

—Dave Marr

A Note to You:

We must watch out for what we're putting on our bodies. I can't believe they let these cancer-causing chemicals in our products. Do these companies even care about our well-being? Can't they come up with a safer option?

Cancer Post #110: Slimming Solutions: January 20th

After my follow-up with my reconstruction surgeon, she released me from all restrictions! I could take off my bra again, my favorite medical release! Ahh, it's the little things. She continued to instruct me on the next phase of my recovery. Massaging my left breast twice daily for the next three months to help soften the hard places created by the radiation. I turned to my husband and gave him a wink, jokingly telling him massaging my breast would be his new job. We both laughed, relieved to have some semblance of normalcy returning to our lives after such a difficult journey.

She asked me, "Do you have any pain or other problems?"

I answered, "Yes. I don't have any pain, but I do have a problem."

With a look of concern, she asked, "What's wrong?"

I sighed and shared my frustration with the doctor. "I've been doing everything right - eating between 1,000 and 1,400 calories daily, walking over 10,000 steps every weekday, and hitting the YMCA thrice weekly for weight-bearing exercises. But despite all of that, I can't seem to lose weight. My body just won't let go of this extra fat."

She studied me with careful eyes and delivered her words with compassion, "Your body has been through a huge hormone adjustment and radiation. Your insulin levels are likely out of balance, making it nearly impossible "for you to shed weight without outside assistance."

My doctor elaborated on the advancements in weight loss medications in recent years. She advised me to speak with my Primary Care Doctor about getting a prescription for one of the available weight loss shots, as they have shown great success. She reassured me that my insurance would likely cover the cost if my doctor wrote the prescription. Interestingly, she also shared that she uses one of the weight loss shots and has seen significant results.

I sent an email to my Primary Care Doctor requesting her to contact my plastic surgeon regarding a solution for my weight problem. I also mentioned in the email that I would be thankful if she could prescribe me this medication because I felt defeated by this weight situation.

Carrying excess weight took a toll on my confidence and self-image. I've come to realize that hiding behind cropped photos on social media isn't the solution.

***

Internet Research:

With growing popularity of new weight loss drugs, doctors emphasize potential risks (msn.com)

Given as daily or weekly injections, these drugs called GLP-1 RAs, help people produce insulin and lower the amount of sugar in the blood. First approved for use in type 2 diabetes patients in 2005 by the U.S. Food and Drug Administration, the medications were quickly noted to promote weight loss.

The FDA, in 2014, later approved a GLP-1 RA for chronic weight management. Additional drugs in the class have since been approved for weight loss.

***

Today's Quote:

"Don't work out because you hate your body — work out because you love it."

—Unknown

A Note to You:

Many pink sisters understand the constant battle with weight that I face. If this isn't an issue for you, I applaud your ability to have control over food. It's tough when food provides instant gratification and comfort, but I hope to overcome it one day. As cancer survivors, we have to be extra mindful of our weight, yet we still struggle. But let's continue to support each other and find strength in our friendship as we work towards healthier habits.

Cancer Post #111: Hand Power: January 23rd

A woman in an online cancer support group shared a valuable tip. Her advice is beneficial for all women, regardless of whether they have cancer or not. She recommended avoiding using a loofa or pouf mesh sponge on our breasts while bathing or showering. Instead, using hands to wash that area, lets us recognize any changes, such as a new lump or bump.

I've always been a faithful sponge user, relying on them to clean and exfoliate my body. But now, after taking the advice of a stranger, I see the value in understanding my body's changes more intimately by using my hands as my washrag. The lady who shared this tip is a genius, pointing out that such a simple change could save your life.

I also researched articles discussing the high levels of bacteria found on washcloths, loofahs, and sponges we use daily. It made me realize our hands are the cleanest option for examining ourselves.

***

Internet Research:

What's Safer to Use in the Shower: Loofah or Washcloth? (oprahdaily.com)

Wait, hands?

That's right! Scrubbing up with your hands is recommended.

"It's best to just wash with our hands," suggests Erum Ilyas, MD, MBE, FAAD. "Loofahs have been well-documented reservoirs of bacteria. They have been shown to grow Pseudomonas, Klebsiella, Enterococcus, Staphylococcus, and more. If you couple the fact that the bacteria are trapped in the fibers of the loofah and that these sponges are used to exfoliate the skin, the risk of infection is much higher. Meanwhile, our hands can be easily cleaned."

***

Today's Quote:

"A bath, a candle, music, and being left alone to soak.... ah."

—Shelley Malicote Stutchman, Author of *PEEK-A-BOOB* and Breast Cancer Survivor

A Note to You:

Sometimes, filling up your tub with warm water and bubbles is just what the doctor ordered. Have you made time for self-care since your diagnosis? It's important to prioritize yourself during this time. Try turning off the lights, lighting candles, and playing soothing music or audiobooks. You could even ask Alexa to play spa music! Take a moment to do a self-breast exam while soaking in the tub. Close your eyes and let all your worries melt away as you focus on taking care of yourself. As the old commercial used to say, "Take me away, Calgon."

Cancer Post #112: Body Dysmorphic Disorder: January 24th

I went to see my primary care doctor. I couldn't wait to start the miracle shot that promised to melt away unwanted pounds. I felt self-conscious in my own body, constantly reminded of the scars on my breast and the daily struggle of wearing a compression sleeve for lymphedema. The Letrozole medication had blocked my estrogen, resulting in fat that gathered in all the wrong places. I wanted to feel pretty!

My doctor informed me my BMI was below the insurance requirement for the shot. She said she would run some lab tests to see if any other medical reason would make me eligible to have insurance cover the medication.

Then she hit me with a bombshell. She claimed I might have body dysmorphic disorder. As I listened, I couldn't help but consider the possibility. Body dysmorphic disorder is a mental health condition that consumes individuals with an irrational obsession over their perceived physical flaws. It's often difficult to diagnose and frequently goes untreated as many sufferers deny its existence within themselves.

During our conversation, my doctor pointed out some statements that indicated body dysmorphia. For example, I shared with her that when I am in the company of other women, I feel like I am the heaviest one in the room. However, I did not disclose to my doctor that when I was growing up, my mother often told me my sister was the pretty one and I was the smart one.

I don't think my mom meant to be mean. She probably believed it would help me concentrate on my studies and work harder to succeed rather than worrying about my looks.

That experience shaped my perception of my appearance and led to a constant desire to be more attractive. Looking back, I wish I had focused on developing my intelligence instead of striving for physical beauty.

Is it possible I have body dysmorphic disorder? Most likely. Even though I knew I should focus on accepting and loving my body, the desire to lose twenty pounds consumed me. Despite this knowledge, I couldn't shake the feeling that shedding those pounds would make me so much happier.

***

Internet Research:

Body Dysmorphic Disorder: Types, Causes, Treatment And More (mantracare.org)

Body dysmorphic disorder is a mental disorder that causes people to have a distorted view of their appearance. They may see themselves as being ugly or deformed, even when they look normal to others. They may avoid social situations or wear clothes that cover up their body. Some people even have surgery to try to fix their perceived flaws. This disorder is just as common in men as in women. It usually starts during the teenage years, but it can also begin later in life.

***

Today's Quote:

"And I said to my body, softly, 'I want to be your friend.' It took a long breath. And replied, 'I have been waiting my whole life for this.'"

—Nayyirah Waheed

A Note to You:

My dear sister, I know the daily battles many of us face with body dysmorphic disorder. The mirror and scale can be our worst enemies, constantly reminding us of our imperfections. But as fellow cancer survivors, we must also recognize and celebrate the strength and resilience of our bodies. We must thank our bodies each day for fighting so hard to overcome such a huge obstacle. So let us start small, appreciating one part of our body at a time - whether it's our fingers holding onto the hand of our loved ones or our legs carrying us to and from numerous doctor's appointments. You are not alone, my sister, and together, we will learn to love and appreciate every inch of ourselves.

NOTES AND THOUGHTS

Chapter Thirty-Six

NO FAVORS

Cancer Post #113: Don't Ask Me: January 30th

If you have a friend or acquaintance going through cancer surgeries and treatments, please refrain from asking them for favors. They are already using all of their strength and resources to battle for their lives. Piling additional burdens or responsibilities on them is not cool.

When I battled through treatments and grappled with both physical and emotional symptoms, I found myself encountering a few requests from others that felt inappropriate. My friends, accustomed to my helpful nature, were used to me going above and beyond for them. Being a people pleaser and caring deeply for my friends' happiness, I often said yes to things even if I didn't want to do them. But during the difficult times of different treatments, my answer had to change. "I'm sorry," I replied with a heavy heart, "but I simply can't."

It was a struggle to prioritize my own well-being and needs over those of others, but it was necessary for my healing journey.

Even after going through cancer treatment, I learned to prioritize my time and energy. So, when a friend approached me, his eyes pleading for help, asked, "Can you spare a hundred dollars? I promise to pay you back within two weeks."

I declined. My bank account was recovering from medical bills, and lending money would add more stress. Turning my friend down hurt my heart, but I knew it was the right decision for my welfare.

I hesitated before answering, my mind racing with excuses and justifications. I couldn't afford to lend any money, not with all the missed work and financial strain. But I hated saying no to a friend in need. Guilt tugged at my conscience as I finally replied, "I'm sorry, I wish I could help, but...I'm just not able to lend any money right now."

He exploded in a fit of rage, hurling piercing insults at me. He told me I was selfish and thought he could count on me. That stung. As the sting of his venomous accusations faded, I saw that this was not a true friend. This person only wanted to take from me and not give anything in return. I learned a valuable lesson. Sometimes, saying no is necessary to weed out the toxic people in our lives.

After overcoming my illness, I took that lesson to heart and transformed it into a source of strength. A close friend confided in me about her overwhelming workload and her concern about finding time to pick up food for an event that evening. Without hesitation, I offered to help by picking up the items she needed. Surprised, she asked, "Why would you do that for me?"

I replied, "Because friends help each other."

I knew the answer to her question from what cancer had taught me. Friendship is about giving, not about getting. I learned the lesson of only being a taker from the friend who asked me for money. I didn't want to be that kind of friend.

During my recovery phase, a fellow member of a group I actively participated in approached me and asked if I could serve as an officer. Although I'm fond of the group and always strive to assist as much as possible, the timing could have been better for such a request. I politely declined, and the individual was understanding. However, the negative response I gave left me feeling down.

Once again, because someone asked a favor of me, I discovered another cancer lesson. At that time, just a few days shy of turning sixty-eight, I had spent years in leadership positions in a variety of organizations. I didn't want to do it anymore. It was my time to go to the events and meetings I chose to attend, relax, and have a good time. I would leave the leadership opportunities to the younger ones. It was their turn to grow and develop and my turn to enjoy and live in the moment.

Another thing that happens when you get diagnosed with cancer is everyone has an opinion on what you should do. When people are diagnosed with cancer, they are bombarded with opinions. Every individual is unique, and what worked for one person may not work for another. I sought out all the information and advice I could find. I've spoken to other cancer survivors who were also overwhelmed by the flood of good intentions. The best approach is to ask if the person wants to hear your perspective and assure that person that you won't be offended if he or she declines. Let people guide the conversation and make their own choices. My friend, if you want to copy this paragraph and post it on your social media so those wanting to give you advice will see it and know how to respond, please do so.

As if dealing with a friend who asked for money wasn't difficult enough, I also had to face hurtful comments from some people who claimed my cancer was a result of my lack of prayer or faith. Those words weighed heavily on me and filled me with guilt and self-doubt. Did my thoughts and actions somehow invite this illness into my body? In search of answers, I turned to a woman I respected, Pastor Laura. With her gentle words and comforting presence, she explained that God does not operate in such vindictive ways. The weight lifted from my shoulders as she reminded me that God's love and grace are unconditional, and my diagnosis was not a punishment or reflection of my worthiness.

This post is a reminder to all those fighting cancer to remember it's okay to say no. This battle consumes your body and mind, and you have every right to protect your limited energy and resources. And for those who have loved ones with cancer, don't demand their involvement or ask them to exert themselves in any way. Show your support through visits, calls, cards, or simply holding their hands. Your robust and energetic friend will be someone you can lean on and depend on again, but just not now.

***

Internet Research:

The Best (and Worst) Ways to Support a Friend with Cancer | Northwestern Medicine

Unhelpful Things to Say to a Person With a Serious Illness

Of course, you would never want to hurt your friend's feelings, but sometimes you might say something that you don't even realize is offensive or insensitive. Here are some general phrases to avoid.

• "I know exactly how you feel." Even if you've experienced a serious illness yourself, you don't know exactly how your friend is feeling, so don't pretend you do. This can make the person feel that their situation is not that big of a deal, when to them, it may be the biggest deal in the world.

• "When (fill in the blank) had this diagnosis, (fill in the blank) happened." The last thing a person with a serious illness wants to hear is someone else's story. You may think you're being helpful or hopeful, but you never know how a person with a serious diagnosis is going to internalize your well-intentioned anecdotes.

• "You're so brave" or "You're so strong." You might think this is an encouraging thing to say to a friend with a serious illness, and maybe in some cases it is. However, telling someone they are brave and strong might pressure them to act differently than they are feeling. While a person with a serious illness might be strong most days, some days they won't be, and that's OK. This also could make them feel like it's their fault if they are not getting better. For example, if they fought harder and were stronger, then they would be getting better. It's unfair to put this undue pressure on them for something that's out of their control.

• "You look different." Or even jokingly saying something like, "Well at least you're losing weight!" Chances are, someone with a serious illness is well aware of how they look, and weight loss (or gain) may not be looked at positively.

• "I'm sure you'll be fine." This may seem like an encouraging, hopeful thing to say, but telling a person with a serious illness that they'll be fine, or telling them not to worry, can be misconstrued as making light of a serious situation. It also promotes a false sense of certainty during an uncertain time. A person with a serious diagnosis should be able to experience feelings like fear and uncertainty, as unpleasant as they may be.

• Questions or statements about time. When a good friend or close family member has a terminal illness, the topic of death might come up, and that's OK. Make sure you follow the person with the terminal illness' lead and ask questions that are appropriate to the conversation.

• "This was God's plan," or "God will take care of it." This oversimplifies the situation and can give the person a false sense of hope. It also can make the person feel like they have no control over what's happening to them.

***

Today's Quote:

"Lots of people want to ride with you in the limo, but what you want is someone who will take the bus with you when the limo breaks down."

—Oprah Winfrey

A friend asked me to share her story. She hopes that you will have a deeper understanding that there will be some people who are cruel to us during this journey. I have copied and pasted her story here.

***

When I was diagnosed with breast cancer in February 2019, I realized some friends and family could possibly pull away from me. I was prepared, but it still hurt and continues to hurt. There have been several incidents which were especially painful. Here is one...

In January 2021, COVID-19 hospitalizations and deaths were going way up and reported daily on television and in newspapers. My husband and I were self-isolating, trying to avoid exposure to COVID-19 - per my oncologist's instructions. I worked from home, we purchased our groceries curbside, and our outings were mostly limited to walks in the neighborhood. Our local hospitals were starting to prioritize care, determining who qualified. I was concerned with my history of cancer and my husband's diabetes; if we got COVID-19, we would get pushed to the back of the line.

At this time, my friend had gone out of town to be with her mother, who had become very ill and then passed. My friend asked me to go to her home and pick up a package off of her porch. I did that. She then asked me to mail it to her. She told me her husband would be in town in two days and he could mail it then, but she wanted to get the package mailed out one day earlier. I explained to my friend that I did not feel comfortable going to the Post Office because of COVID-19 and apologized.

My friend intended to text her husband, but she texted me instead. Apparently, she was angry with me that I would not go to the Post Office for her so she could get the package one day sooner. My friend wrote, "She voted for Biden...Forget policy differences. I hope she enjoys cancer treatment on Obamacare and worse."

I was heartbroken.

In April 2022, I was diagnosed with breast cancer again, so I had a double mastectomy, but I am doing fine and enjoying life.

***

A Note to You:

My Pink Sisters, cancer teaches us countless lessons, some of them bittersweet. You may lose friends on this journey, but you will also gain new ones who will support you through thick and thin. Perhaps the most important lesson is learning to say no. Take a deep breath and confidently declare, "No, I cannot (fill in the blank)." It's okay to put yourself first and prioritize your own well-being during this difficult time. Remember, you are strong and capable and will emerge from this with a newfound sense of empowerment. Stay resilient, my dear survivor sister.

NOTES AND THOUGHTS

Chapter Thirty-Seven

HAPPY BIRTHDAY

Cancer Post #114: Joyous Anniversary of Birth: February 3rd

The news of my cancer diagnosis last February left me unsure if I would make it to my next birthday. But as time passed, I realized I would indeed conquer this disease.

I celebrated my birthday today, reveling in the feeling of being alive. It was a glorious and sweet sensation. I basked in the flood of birthday wishes on my Facebook page, and my heart exploded with gratitude. As I read each message, I sent vibes of good health and happiness to every person who had taken the time to reach out. Images of their smiling faces filled me with pleasure.

I indulged in a heavenly angel food cake, drenched in a rich chocolate sauce and topped with homemade whipped cream. Every bite was a symphony of flavors, each one crafted by the skilled hands of my friend and professional baker, Pam. As we savored the decadent dessert, I raised my glass of Silver Oak, my favorite exquisite wine, in a toast to the gratitude of another birthday. Surrounded by my closest friends Ron and Luana and my loving husband Neil, this birthday celebration was perfect. And what better way to continue than with a luxurious dinner at an upscale steakhouse? The tender cuts of meat and the warm, lively conversation made for a five-star experience. When the evening ended, I vowed to always indulge in dessert first.

Reflecting on the grace of reaching my sixty-eighth birthday filled me with profound gratitude. Despite occasional grumbling about getting older, the battle against cancer this year imbued each day with a preciousness beyond measure. The love exchanged with my cherished friends and family has been a true balm to my soul. While some may find this post sentimental, every word springs forth from the depths of my heart.

***

Internet Research:

Celebrating Healthy Birthdays - (integrativeoncology-essentials.com)

For many people who have survived cancer, birthdays take on a whole new meaning. They're not just an occasion to celebrate their birth but also a chance to give thanks that they're still alive – sometimes, against poor odds. For the nearly 12 million cancer survivors currently living in the U.S., staying healthy and celebrating as many birthdays as possible is the number one goal.

***

Today's Quote:

"God gave us the gift of life; it is up to us to give ourselves the gift of living well."

—Voltaire

A Note to You:

My friend, when your special day draws near, I'm grateful you get to celebrate another year of new adventures. Find a way to bring happiness into your world on your birthday. It could be an extravagant party, an intimate get-together with those dear to you, or a peaceful day dedicated to self-nurturing. Take a pause to explore the depths of your feelings as you commemorate another important achievement after beating cancer. Have the most joyous birthday, my Pink Sister. Remember to savor a slice of cake for me.

Cancer Post #115: Nervous: February 6th

When the day of my one-year follow-up approached, I felt a sense of apprehension. The memory of my last yearly mammogram, once a mere routine appointment, now haunted me. That fateful call summoning me back for further examinations replayed in my mind. Now, as I readied myself to confront this milestone, anxiety flooded my emotions.

Even though my instincts told me I was overreacting, the fear of another tumor gnawed at me. I didn't feel I had the strength to endure all this again. In desperation, I prayed to God, hoping that he would hear my pleas and spare me from going through such a grueling experience once more. I hoped God was listening.

***

Internet Research:

Coping With Scanxiety During Cancer Treatment (verywellhealth.com)

Scanxiety is the term that's been coined to describe the anxiety people with cancer feel while waiting for scans. Whether scans are being done for diagnosis, to monitor treatment, to check for a recurrence, or simply for follow-up, it doesn't matter. It's scary to wait.

We know there is anxiety with having scans, and that it's the rule rather than the exception. Research even tells us that it doesn't really matter what we think the results of our scans will be. There could be a 99 percent chance that it will be good or a 99 percent chance that it will be bad news. Even if our chances lie on the good side, our brains (and whatever goes on to release stress hormones in our bodies) don't seem to register those numbers.

***

Today's Quote:

"Giving in to the darkness offers no benefit."

—Marivel Preciado

A Note for You:

I wondered how long this scanxiety lasts. I've asked other cancer survivors, and they all tell me the same thing, "A lifetime."

It's hard for anyone who hasn't been through it to understand the lasting effects of PTSD we experience. But you get it, don't you? That feeling of dread every time another follow-up comes around. If you need someone by your side during these appointments, reach out. And should you catch sight of another facing these trials alone, extend your hand as a beacon of understanding. Through shared journeys and outstretched hands, we can navigate the labyrinth of fears that threaten to consume us. The best way to overcome our fears is to reach out to others.

/ # NOTES AND THOUGHTS

Chapter Thirty-Eight
INTIMATE POSTS

Cancer Post #116: Potentially Controversial: February 8th

These final posts have been carefully guarded and saved for the conclusion of this book, as their contents are intimate and potentially controversial.

Revealed within these final pages are my raw emotions - moments of acceptance, rage, resentment, gratitude, tranquility, and anxiousness. After receiving the news of a clear follow-up mammogram, I felt determined to strive towards becoming the strongest and most resilient version of myself - Shelley reborn.

I'm grateful cancer taught me valuable lessons I needed to learn. I've stopped blaming myself for past mistakes and learned to appreciate my family, husband, and friends. Each morning, when I wake up, I try to look at the world with a fresh perspective and a bigger heart. I've also discovered I can say no. During my journey, I've had moments where I've struggled with my faith and questioned the path that God placed me. But I've concluded that God gave me the words and skills to write this book to help others, so I'm no longer angry, but indebted for the journey that brought me here.

The advancements in breast cancer treatment have filled me with excitement. However, our current methods are still archaic and brutal. I hope to witness the eradication of cancer during my lifetime and see the development of more gentle and efficient treatments. My ultimate dream is for more discoveries to be made in preventing cancer through nutrition and supplements.

Sitting at my cluttered desk, fingers flying over the keyboard as I finished these final posts, I took a moment to savor the steam rising from my mug of freshly brewed coffee. The rich aroma of hot coffee mingled with the sweet creaminess of two tablespoons of half and half, delighted my senses. Each sip a small moment of indulgence, a reward for hard work. Reflecting on the past year, every experience took on a new level of meaning and gratitude, from moving into a new home and getting married to an unforgettable honeymoon. Even facing a partial mastectomy and undergoing brachytherapy and reconstruction. The year was a rollercoaster ride of emotions and experiences. I'm grateful for my new pink sister friends who have supported me every step of the way. As I took in the warmth of my coffee and the comfort of my surroundings, I was reminded to cherish each moment, no matter how challenging or unexpected.

***

Internet Research:

Breast Cancer Cure: Are We Close, Research, and More (healthline.com)

Scientists continue to conduct clinical trials to develop and test treatments for breast cancer.

These trials may help them develop new treatment options and learn which types of people are most likely to benefit from available treatments. Over time, this might lead to more effective and personalized treatment plans.

***

Today's Quote:

"The most important aim of cancer treatment is to achieve cure and secondly life prolongation and relief of sufferings. We must understand the mechanisms of how cancer develops and progresses to unlock new ways to prevent, detect and treat it."

—Dr. Dinesh Kacha – Researcher

A Note to You:

We, the survivors who have battled cancer, have a duty to future generations. We must do everything in our power to find a cure. Whether it's participating in clinical trials or walking for hours at fundraisers, we must not back down from this fight. Let's also raise our voices to the government, demanding more funding for research. I took part in an online study on the emotional impact of cancer, and not only did I possibly help others, but it gave me insight into my own journey. My fellow fighters, let's unite and end breast cancer once and for all so that our daughters and granddaughters never have to experience its devastation.

Cancer Post #117: My Son Has Cancer: February 9th

In 2021, before I had done any research about cancer my phone rang, etched in my memory was my son's voice, usually warm and vibrant, was now strained and weak. "Mom," he stuttered out, "I just left the doctor's office...they found cancer. In my prostate."

The news hit me like a ton of bricks, every mother's worst nightmare come true. My sweet son battling a life-threatening illness.

My son Ryan, my pride and joy, made a decision about his cancer treatment. After hours of consulting with his doctor and wife, they settled on a wait-and-watch approach. My heart was heavy with conflicting emotions - on one hand, I desperately wanted him to do everything in his power to get rid of the cancer, but on the other hand, I could understand his concerns about potential side effects from a prostatectomy. As much as I longed to take control and protect him as his mother, I knew he was now an adult, and it was ultimately his decision. I could only offer my unwavering support and respect for whatever path he chose to take.

As parents, his dad and I were shattered by our son's diagnosis. Our hearts felt like they had been broken into a million tiny pieces. Ryan, our Little King, was facing a fierce battle against cancer. We made a solemn vow to each other: we would stop at nothing to help him fight this war. Horace, his dad, became consumed with research on Ryan's condition and the best course of action. He spoke directly with the urologist, uncovering Ryan's decision to forgo surgery for his cancerous cluster was actually the cutting-edge approach. Each new piece of information brought us closer to understanding and supporting Ryan in his brave fight.

Desperate tears streamed down my face as I begged the heavens above. "Please, God," I pleaded, "if someone must suffer from cancer on this earth, let it be me instead of my son."

I offered myself up as a sacrifice, willing to endure any amount of agony and suffering if it meant sparing my child from his illness.

A year passed, and I received my diagnosis of breast cancer. Fear crashed over me, but deep down, a strange sense of relief settled in my heart. In some twisted way, I felt like it was God's plan for me to take on Ryan's cancer and relieve him of his burden. However, when we received the results of Ryan's one-year follow-up, it became clear this wasn't the case. Ryan's cancer remained, stubbornly refusing to let go of its grip on him.

The foundation of my faith crumbled beneath my feet, leaving me feeling adrift and shattered. How could this happen? Not only did I have cancer, but Ryan's cancer didn't disappear. In a moment of vulnerability, I opened up to someone about my plea to God to save my son, hoping for comfort and understanding. Instead, I was met with harsh judgment and accusations. According to the person I shared with, I also got cancer because I invited evil into my body by making a deal with God, and the cancer was my divine punishment. The very idea made bile rise in my throat and tears sting my eyes.

Grappling with the lashing I had received, still needing to understand, I reached out to other friends with strong faith. Their unwavering conviction sparked a glimmer of hope within me, and they gently explained that God's ways were not always easily understood. And so, every day, I prayed for my son, hoping my words were heard. I prayed, humbled and broken, and peace and comfort filled my heart. I suddenly felt God or the Universe understood the boundless love of a mother's heart for her son.

***

Internet Research:

Detroit Baptist Theological Seminary "God, if You...then I'll...": Why You Can't Barter with God - Detroit Baptist Theological Seminary (dbts.edu)

Why does it matter whether or not we can barter with God? Because if we can't barter with Him, that means we have to accept His terms. We can't entice Him with our offers. We can only accept His offers.

***

Today's Quote:

"If I had to choose between loving my child and breathing, I would use my last breath to tell you I love you."

—Unknown

A Note to You:

Years ago, I sat by my mother-in-law's side as she lost not one but two of her beloved children to the unforgiving grip of cancer. Despite the heart-wrenching pain and endless tears, her unwavering faith and strength shone through like a beacon of hope in the darkest of times. Now, as I navigate my own son's battle with this ruthless disease, I finally understand the depth of her anguish. My heart aches for any of you reading this who has had to endure the agony of watching your child suffer. As we hold on tightly to one another, our arms forming a protective shield against the pain, I am reminded of the power of love and support. Hugs, my Pink Sisters.

… PEEK-A-BOOB

NOTES AND THOUGHTS

CHAPTER THIRTY-NINE

MUSIC AND WORDS

Cancer Post #118: Music of Joel Sebring: March 4th

Occasionally, blessings from God or the universe cross our paths. As a lover of music, I often asked Alexa to play my favorite songs to distract me from the pain of cancer and my inflamed joints. One day, as I scrolled through Facebook, I stumbled upon a post by a talented singer based in Nashville, Joel Sebring. At first, I wondered if he was related to a kind gentleman with the same last name who had volunteered for Hospice with me. Although I discovered he wasn't, my interest in this artist sparked like wildfire. And let me tell you, his pictures were eye-catching! I even had a hot flash from the excitement while looking at them.

As I scrolled through Joel's Facebook posts, a sense of warmth and positivity filled my heart. There was something about him that just radiated goodness. And when I would feel overwhelmed by the brutal effects of cancer treatment, his music became my refuge. Each strum of his guitar, each note from his voice, offered healing powers beyond what any pain pill could offer. His lyrics spoke directly to my soul, and his melodies danced through my body, easing the tension and pain. In those moments, Joel's music became more than just a source of comfort - it was a lifeline.

I left a few comments on Joel's Facebook page. I couldn't believe it when he responded back. He often answered with a simple heart symbol or a genuine reply. The fact that this successful, attractive, and incredibly talented musician took the time to interact with his fans only made me admire him more. I felt grateful for the connection we had through social media.

Growing up on the farm, I thought I had everything I could ever want. But growing older, I began to question my place in this insular world. While my childhood was filled with joys like helping my dad and spending time with my much-loved animals, there was also a sense of restlessness within me. And that's where Joel's music came in - his country-soul fusion spoke to me.

When I was uncertain if cancer would claim me as its next victim, the melody and lyrics of "Fly Angel Fly" echoed through my mind. Each note reminded me of the fragility of life and the looming threat of death. I found solace in the lyrics - a promise that even if my body failed me, my spirit would soar freely like an angel, released from the physical torment of cancer. And now, as I emerge victorious from this battle, that song will forever be etched into my heart as a reminder of strength and resilience.

The tune of Joel's song, "I'll Be Fine," resonated with me on a deeper level. With each verse, I replaced the lyrics about a broken relationship with my own struggles with cancer. The song reminded me I would be fine even when my body was weak and failing. Music has a powerful way of connecting us to our emotions and reminding us of our resilience. I'm grateful for empowering songs that lift people's spirits and give them the courage to keep fighting.

The song "I Knew" is a love song that made my heart smile. It's because I knew that my husband, Neil, would never leave me. He's stood by me through every cancer surgery and treatment and all the days that I had no energy. Whenever I looked into Neil's eyes, I knew.

Joel's song, "Say A Prayer for Me," brings to light the suffering of those less fortunate than ourselves. It serves as a reminder that, despite our own struggles, we are fortunate to have a roof over our heads, food on the table, and a support system to lean on. This song has the power to shift our focus away from our own problems and toward the needs of others - those who are homeless, broken, and struggling. The lyrics are powerful, and they call us to action.

Sometimes, when you want to hear a good beat, a song that makes you want to wiggle your booty, Joel's "There Goes My Heart Again" is a perfect choice. Walking is a great way to build back your strength after all the breast cancer treatments, and this song will put pep into your step.

***

Internet Research:

https://www.webmd.com/breast-cancer/ss/slideshow-surprising-breast-cancer-hel

Listening to your favorite tunes has probably helped you get over a breakup or power through a workout. This ability to connect you to your feelings is why music can also help during treatment. Studies show a program with a trained music therapist can drop pain levels, improve state of mind, and reduce worry for people with breast cancer.

***

Today's Quote:

"Rock on, Rockstar."

—Joel Sebring

A Note to You:

Remember how music bonds you to so many people and special times? Music has this incredible way of calming our minds and touching our hearts like nothing else can. And during your tough times, when the pain of cancer physically and emotionally feels endless, turn on some music to help ease your pain and fears. So why not try something new? Explore a new artist and follow them on social media; who knows where it could lead? Joel's Sebring's music is groovy and worth a listen. Who knows what you might discover when you go on a musical journey!

Cancer Post #119: Unraveling Meanings: March 5th

Cancer has its own set of specialized terminology. Here are a few keywords to help understand and differentiate it.

Warrior: Someone currently in treatment for cancer.

Thriver: Someone living with stage 4 cancer.

Survivor: Someone who has finished and survived treatment.

Tumor: Abnormal or excessive tissue growth. Tumors can be benign, precancerous, or cancerous.

Node Negative: This means that the cancer has not spread to the lymph nodes.

Indolent Cancer: A cancer that grows very slowly.

Malignant: This word, in conjunction with cancer, means that the diagnosis is not benign but cancerous.

Cancer: A disease characterized by abnormal cell growth in an organ or organ system that may spread to other parts of the body. There are more than 100 types of cancer.

Biopsy: A procedure in which a piece of tissue is removed from the body to be analyzed in a lab. A biopsy is often preformed to determine if a tumor is malignant. Only a piece of the concerning tissue is removed with a needle.

BRCA1 and BRCA2: The names of two genes that, when mutated, increase the risk of breast and ovarian cancers, as well as others, such as prostate cancer, pancreatic cancer, and skin cancer. These can be passed down through families and are more prevalent in certain ethnic communities.

Cancer-Related Lymphedema: Lymphedema is a condition that causes swelling, mostly in the arms or legs but also in the face, neck, belly, and genitals. It happens when lymph fluid builds up under the skin, which can occur when the lymphatic system is disrupted or blocked. Cancer and certain cancer therapies, like surgery, radiation, and chemotherapy, can affect the flow of lymph fluid and lead to lymphedema. This is known as "cancer-related lymphedema."

Carcinoma: Carcinoma refers to cancers that develops from epithelial cells that line inner or outer surfaces of tissues and blood vessels.

Chemotherapy: Anti-cancer drugs, usually used in combination, that treat cancer.

Cold Cap: A hat that's filled with a chilled gel coolant and worn to help prevent women from losing some of their hair during chemotherapy. It works by narrowing the blood vessels beneath the skin of the scalp so less chemo reaches the hair follicle. The cold also lowers the activity of the hair follicles. The cap is worn before, during, and after chemo treatments.

Expanders: These inflatable breast implants are used after a mastectomy is performed and are designed to stretch the skin and muscle to make room for permanent implants. During a mastectomy, plastic surgeons insert tissue expanders beneath the skin and chest muscle. The expanders are gradually enlarged by filling them with periodic injections of saltwater solution over several weeks or months. This helps stretch the area and prepare it for an implant.

Hormone Therapy: Also known as endocrine therapy, this form of treatment is used to treat cancers that rely on hormones to grow, such as breast and prostate cancer. It uses agents that block the body's ability to produce hormones or interfere with how hormones function within the body.

Lumpectomy: Surgery to remove cancer from a breast in which the tumor and a margin of some surrounding tissue is removed, but a large part of the breast is left intact.

Lymph Nodes: Small ovoid-shaped structures located throughout the body, concentrated in the neck, underarm, chest, belly, and groin, that filter harmful substances out of the lymphatic system. Lymph nodes contain immune cells that assist in fighting infection.

Margin: When a surgeon removes cancerous tissue from the body, they will remove a span of normal tissue surrounding the tumor – the margin- to make sure all cancerous tissue has been excised.

Mastectomy: Surgery to remove the entire breast.

Metastasis: Metastasis has occurred when cancer cells have spread from the site of origin to a secondary or distant site in the body.

Adjuvant-therapy: Adjuvant therapy is a secondary method of treatment that is performed after the primary treatment method to lower the risk of the cancer returning. Examples include: chemotherapy and radiation therapy.

Adverse Events: Adverse events are also known as side effects. An adverse event is an unexpected or dangerous reaction to a treatment or medication. They are captured in the clinical trial and should be reported as part of the safety profile of the treatment.

Axillary Lymph Node Dissection: Lymph nodes are small glands located in the underarm area. When someone's lymph nodes are removed the procedure is called an axillary lymph node dissection. This surgery is usually combined with a mastectomy.

Biomarker: Also known as a molecular marker, a biomarker can be proteins, gene mutations, gene rearrangements, extra copies of genes, missing genes or other molecules that can affect how cancer cells grow, multiply, die and respond to other compounds in the body. Biomarkers can be found in the blood, tissue and other body fluids and can be used to help identify to which treatment the cancer may respond.

EBC: Early Breast Cancer EBC is breast cancer that is contained in the breast. It has been detected before it's spread to the lymph nodes or the armpit.

Estrogen Receptor Positive: Estrogen Receptor Positive (ER+) is used to describe breast cancer cells that may receive signals from the hormone estrogen to promote their growth.

HER2: In HER2-positive patients, your cancer cells make an excess amount of the HER2 protein. Originally made to control a breast cell's growth, when the HER2 protein doesn't work properly, breast cells can overproduce. This breast cancer tends to be aggressive, but there have been important breakthroughs in treatment.

ILC (Invasive Lobular Carcinoma): ILC (or invasive lobular carcinoma) is a type of breast cancer that starts in the milk-producing lobules of the breast and has spread to surrounding breast tissue. It is the second most common type of breast cancer, next to IDC (invasive ductal carcinoma).

NED ("No Evidence of Disease"): NED is a term used when tests show no presence of cancer cells in someone who was previously being treated for cancer. NED has replaced the term remission because it is more accurate.

Situ: Situ is used to describe a tumor, cancer, etc. which is confined to where it first started. In other words, it hasn't spread. For example, ductal carcinoma in situ, is a breast cancer found in the milk ducts, which has not spread to other tissues or parts of the body.

***

Internet Research:

Why is cancer called cancer? | Metro News

What are the origins of the word cancer?

The origin of the word cancer can be traced back to the 'Father of Medicine' Greek physician Hippocrates (460-370 BC).

Hippocrates used the terms carcinos and carcinoma to describe non-ulcer forming and ulcer-forming tumors.

The Roman physician, Celsus (28-50 BC), later translated the Greek term into cancer.

***

Today's Quote:

"Overcoming cancer awakens a courage and confidence inside of you that makes you want to live big, bold and intentional every day. It becomes much easier to grow as a person, because you have already been forced way out of your comfort zone. I don't worry about failing when I try new things now, because my inner voice always reminds me that 'this' can't be any harder than cancer!"

—Renee Ward

A Note to You:

As you navigate this cancer journey, you're bombarded with unfamiliar words that seem like a foreign language. But don't let them pass through one ear and out the other. They could hold vital information that no one has taken the time to explain to you. Look them up online or stop anyone, even a doctor, in their tracks and demand they define any terms you don't understand. And remember, my dear friend, amidst all this confusion and fear, there is one thing that needs no explanation: we pink sisters are here to love you through this experience.

NOTES AND THOUGHTS

Chapter Forty

RECURRENCE

Cancer Post #120: Stand by your Friend: March 27th

When I read Jodi's post, my heart dropped. She shared that her latest mammogram revealed a spot, later confirmed by an ultrasound and MRI. Jodi radiated beauty and Hollywood glamour and always showed boundless generosity and kindness. It made me question why this had to happen to someone like her. Why did it have to be Jodi?

The doctor's words were foreboding. "It's not really a mass," he said, using clinical terms like 'architectural distortion.'

For a brief moment, Jodi clung to a glimmer of hope. But as soon as she looked up the meaning of those words, her heart sank. Architectural distortion is a twisting or bending of the breast tissue with no definite lump visible. It could be a sign of something malignant or benign, and she prayed for the latter. However, her research revealed that 74.5% of cases involving architectural distortions turned out to be cancerous. The weight of this statistic settled on her shoulders like a 2-ton anvil.

Jodi drummed her fingers against the armrest of her chair; she had been through this before, with endless waiting. But this time, it felt even more cruel and frustrating. The doctor's office was supposed to call her to schedule her next round of testing, but her phone remained silent. She felt like no one cared. Determined not to let them keep her in the dark, Jodi decided to call them the following morning. She needed answers.

I took Jodi to lunch, and part of me wanted to broach the topic and offer my support, while another part feared pushing her too far and causing more pain. Should I bring up the pending diagnosis or stick to a light conversation? However, Jodi, being Jodi, led the conversation, and we discussed her hopes and fears of what the results would show.

Our hearts raced, and our minds filled with dread as Jodi went back for further testing. The fear of a cancer recurrence loomed like a shadow over our breast cancer community. But when the results came back negative for cancer, we all let out a collective sigh of relief. Jodi was more than a survivor - she was a leader, an inspiration to us all. And if cancer ever dared to rear its ugly head again, it would have faced an army of fierce women ready to stand by her side and fight alongside her until victory was won.

***

Internet Research:

Reducing the Risk of Breast Cancer Recurrence (verywellhealth.com)

Before talking about measures that may help lower recurrence risk, it's important to not add to the stigma of the disease. Some people do absolutely everything right and their breast cancer recurs anyway. Similarly, some people eat poorly, smoke, and drink heavily and their cancer never recurs. While you may be able to decrease your risk of recurrence to a degree, dealing with breast cancer is dealing with a mutated clone of cells that doesn't think or follow the rules.

***

Today's Quote:

"Here's to you—I hope that you get steadier, stronger, and better every day."

—Unknown

A Note to You:

It's terrifying to hear about a friend or someone in your support group having a breast cancer recurrence. It reminds us how fragile life can be and how we must remain vigilant against this disease. But don't let fear make you back away from your friends. Just being there for them, offering support and love, means more than you know. And if you struggle to cope with the news, don't hesitate to seek counseling. We all hope and pray never to face this battle again, but we must always be prepared for it. Let's continue to support each other and stay strong together in this fight against breast cancer. Blessings to us all.

SHELLEY MALICOTE STUTCHMAN

NOTES AND THOUGHTS

Chapter Forty-One
DOWN AND DIRTY

Cancer Post #121: Sexy Challenges: March 29th

Why is the topic of intimacy rarely discussed with doctors when it comes to breast cancer? Intimacy issues can become a primary concern for couples and can even lead to the dissolution of marriages. For many couples, sexual activity is an essential aspect of their relationship, and changes after a breast cancer diagnosis can be challenging to navigate. Unfortunately, many couples suffer in silence as doctors rarely address the changes that occur in the bedroom once a patient is diagnosed with breast cancer.

Here is my sex story:

As soon as the word "cancer" was spoken, my whole being changed. No longer was I a carefree, adventurous senior citizen in the bedroom. All I could think about was my diagnosis and what would happen next. I lost all sense of fun and spontaneity. Physically, nothing had changed - I still responded to his touch and craved intimacy. But I had no spunk to be creative or exciting in bed.

Then came the partial mastectomy and removal of two lymph nodes. After the surgery, and before I could even peak at the outcome of what was left of my breast, a tight surgical bra covered every inch of my chest. Let me share with you that surgical bras are not the least bit sexy. The doctor told me to wait several weeks before the dressings and bra came off. She also said no sex for six weeks.

As the big day approached, when we could be intimate again, we both felt a sense of fear and uncertainty. He was worried about causing me pain if he touched me or putting his weight on me, while I was anxious about him finding me unattractive. But after working through our concerns, he reassured me he still found me beautiful, and I assured him that it was okay to touch me. I would let him know if it hurt. The only significant change in our sexual encounters at this point was in my own perception; I felt ugly when I was naked.

The next step in my treatment was radiation. Because of the tubes implanted in my breast for the radiation seeds to travel through, sex was off-limits during this time. The treatments left me exhausted, and I worried about being radioactive. I didn't want to do anything that might cause cancer in Neil. He never admitted it, but I think he was a little worried about kissing my nipples and the effects of radiation. In an earlier chapter I mentioned when I asked my doctor, "If my husband kissed my nipple, was there a risk of transferring radioactivity to him?"

She assured me there was no danger of that happening, and she also commended me for asking the question, as she had never thought to bring up the topic of sex and radiation therapy herself. It's a shame we must gather our bravery to ask these types of questions instead of being fully informed by our doctors.

Just six days after my final radiation treatment, Neil and I stood hand in hand at the altar and exchanged vows. Our wedding was a groovy, 70s-themed party filled with music, laughter, and love. It was a celebration of not only our marriage but also my victory over cancer. We set off for our honeymoon two days later, eager to start our new life together. As we made love during those first few nights as husband and wife, it was tender and gentle, full of unspoken understanding and deep affection. The passion between us still burned strong, but I lacked the stamina to be the same wild and adventurous lover I once was.

When we returned from our honeymoon, my doctor handed me a small bottle of pills with strict instructions: one every morning. She warned me about potential joint pain, but she didn't mention the other side effects. My libido vanished without estrogen, making intimacy with my husband feel like a painful chore. The hormone blockers drained every ounce of energy from my body, leaving me exhausted and barely able to function. And the dryness…it felt like shards of glass were piercing my insides whenever we tried to be intimate, even with lubrication. What a spiteful side effect.

Despite our age and experience, my husband and I struggled to find a new normal for sex. He remained patient and never pressured me, but I couldn't help feeling like I wasn't sexy anymore. I wondered how different things would be if we were a young couple in this situation. It would be a living hell for them, constantly struggling to keep up with each other's expectations and desires.

In a previous post, I revealed the reasons behind my decision to stop taking the hormone blocker. And now, as my body begins to produce its own lubrication again, a sense of relief and longing flooded me. The wetness was less, but the pleasure was back, and my sexual appetite was reignited for my beloved husband. Yet, despite all this, there lies a void within me - the wild, carefree side that used to revel in passion and adventure. It remains elusive, suffocated by the weight of self-doubt. Perhaps it's my age catching up with me. Or maybe it's the constant reminder that my body is no longer what it once was.

Our sex life is far from over. In fact, I can't wait to retire and have even more time and energy for intimacy. We set a goal to keep the passion alive and thriving. Maybe that's a goal I'll be able to keep. It's with the anticipation of my retirement that I can give him that look that we are about to have a romp in the bedroom. Once I can retire, that action can happen in the middle of the afternoon on a school day.

The topic of sex and breast cancer remains largely unspoken, shrouded in a veil of societal taboos, and overshadowed by the primary focus of cancer treatment - getting rid of the disease and preventing its return. However, a part of me, my inner wild child, is again emerging and reclaiming my sense of self, urging me to open up about this crucial aspect of life that is often ignored.

***

Internet Research:

How Cancer and Cancer Treatment Can Affect Sexuality | American Cancer Society

Sex, sexuality, and intimacy are just as important for people with cancer as they are for people who don't have cancer. In fact, sexuality and intimacy have been shown to help people face cancer by helping them deal with feelings of distress, and when going through treatment. But the reality is that a person's sex organs, sexual desire (sex drive or libido), sexual function, well-being, and body image can be affected by cancer and cancer treatment. How a person shows sexuality can also be affected.

Today's Quote:

"Sex: the thing that takes up the least amount of time and causes the most amount of trouble."

—John Barrymore

A Note to You:

When I told my oncologist I was writing this book, she asked me this question, "Will you please include a section on sex? I know we doctors get so focused on beating the cancer we don't always provide our patients enough information on this topic."

Check out the Facebook group "Sex after Breast Cancer." It's an excellent resource for tips and support from other women who have gone through similar experiences.

And speaking of lifesavers, I've personally found these hormone-free products to be helpful: Key-E suppositories provide your vaginal area with the Vitamin E it needs and acts as a lubricant. These can be purchased on Amazon and run around $15.73 for ten suppositories. Revaree is a very good moisturizer with Hyaluronic Acid. Hyaluronic Acid effectively delivers moisturizing benefits. You can also purchase these on Amazon. They are pricy at $67.00 for ten. I recommend alternating the Vitamin E with the Revaree. I use it twice a week and have regained the moisture in my vaginal area.

Don't be shy about using a vibrator. This toy has helped me get back in touch with my sexuality and pleasure.

Please don't be embarrassed as you find a new normal for your sex life. Find what works for you and your partner, or what brings you pleasure by yourself. We were created with sexual desires. Let's not let cancer take away our sexy selves.

PEEK-A-BOOB

NOTES AND THOUGHTS

Chapter Forty-Two

LITTLE GIRL'S THOUGHTS ABOUT BREAST CANCER

Cancer Post #122: Little Girls Are Listening: April 11th

I recently discovered something important that I feel the need to share. When discussing breast cancer in the presence of young girls, we must be cautious and mindful of our language and phrasing.

A devastating blow struck the mother of an eleven-year-old when she received a diagnosis of breast cancer. With determination, she underwent a double mastectomy and endured all subsequent treatments and medications. This wasn't her family's first encounter with this battle - her mother had also been diagnosed with breast cancer, going through the same process of a double mastectomy and tough treatments.

In the brightly lit bathroom, the little girl peered at herself in the mirror. Two small bumps had sprouted on her chest overnight, and she felt both fascinated and horrified. Her mother gently explained to her daughter she needed to start wearing a bra. The little girl stubbornly refused, crossing her arms over her chest. After some tears and tantrums, her mom finally convinced her to go bra shopping at Target, promising to make it a fun and exciting experience.

The morning after the shopping excursion, the mother discovered the bras in the trash can. She couldn't understand why her daughter threw them away. Did her daughter hate them? Or maybe they didn't fit properly? She confronted her daughter, "Why did you throw the bras away?"

The little girl's developing frame shook with rage as she stomped, refusing to utter a single word. Grandma came over to help figure out why her granddaughter reacted like this to her new bras. Grandma sat on the edge of the little girl's bed, wrapping her arms around her granddaughter. She gently brought up the topic of bras, and the little girl burst into tears. Grandma held her close, comfortingly whispering words of reassurance. As the sobs subsided, the little girl finally confided in her grandmother, "I don't want my breasts, Grandma. You and Mama both said they almost killed you. I'm scared they'll do the same to me."

There are many sayings and quotes about your breasts almost killing you, and most of us say them for comic relief. There is a T-shirt you can buy that has printed on it, "Yes, these are fake; my real ones tried to kill me."

It's crucial that we carefully choose our words when discussing breast cancer with young, developing girls. They are always listening, absorbing every word we say. These precious, innocent souls are fearful of witnessing their own mother or grandmother battling this disease. I never truly grasped the weight of our words in shaping their perceptions until I heard this mother share her story about her daughter.

With a gentle insistence, Grandma and the little girl retrieved the discarded bras from the trash. She encouraged the girl to put them away in her drawer and wear them when comfortable. A few days later, the little girl wore her bras without fanfare or fuss from her mother or grandmother. They wanted to normalize this stage of her development.

***

Internet Research:

Are the kids all right? When breast cancer runs in the family - CBS News

A new study of more than 800 girls and their mothers - from families with and without a history of breast cancer or a known genetic risk for it - found that girls from breast cancer families have higher levels of anxiety about their risk for the disease. Their general emotional well-being, though, was no different than that of their peers from families without the disease.

***

Today's Quote:

"An individual doesn't get cancer, a family does."

—Terry Tempest Williams

A Note to You:

When I heard this woman's personal journey with her daughter, I realized the impact of my words on children. Let's be mindful of our language when we're in the company of young girls and respect their innocence, as it can shape their perception of this important issue.

Chapter Forty-Three

THE CRUISE

Cancer Post #123: Seafaring: April 24th

The sibling cruise that was once on my bucket list is now checked off as completed.

My two biological children, Ginger and Ryan, and my bonus children, Melissa and Natalie, had a great time aboard the Royal Caribbean. I uploaded our vacation photos on Facebook and wrote this comment, "Without cancer, I would never have gone on this cruise because I used to believe there was always another day. I'm grateful cancer opened my eyes."

My friend, Becky, replied, "Instead of being grateful for cancer, be grateful that your eyes were opened."

Becky's words ring true, resonating deep within me. I never could have imagined that cancer would be the catalyst for opening my eyes to truly living. The disease, with all its pain and struggle, gifted me with a new perspective on life. I am grateful for every moment and memory, eagerly embracing each day with a hunger to experience as much as possible before the sun sets. Cancer may have brought darkness into my life. Still, it also brought a newfound appreciation for the brightness and beauty of every passing moment.

The cruise was the perfect vacation for our group. With excitement, we planned out our days on board - some of us eager to relax by the pool and feel the ocean breeze, while others looked forward to late nights full of fun activities. However, we all made a promise to have dinner together every evening, allowing everyone their own time during the day. This simple agreement brought us all closer as we shared stories and laughter over delicious meals each night. Whether we were lounging or exploring, the cruise provided endless options for a perfect vacation with our group.

The memory of my second chance at life is burned into my mind, a precious gift I will never forget. I'm committed to living with an unrelenting fire that consumes any doubt or hesitation, driving me toward a fearless existence. I hope the same for you.

***

Internet Research:

https://www.asbestos.com/blog/2013/10/15/cancer-patient-caregiver-vacation-cruise

Remember that this is a vacation. Let go of some of your worries and enjoy this special time together. Happy Cruising.

***

Today's Quote:

"Twenty years from now, you will be more disappointed by the things you didn't do than those you did. So, throw off the bowlines. Sail away from safe harbor. Catch the wind in your sails. Explore. Dream. Discover."

—Mark Twain

A Note to You:

My dear pink sisters, thank you for reading this book and sharing my journey. I've written this book from the perspective of my personal experience with breast cancer. Whether we've shared the same stages and treatments or not, our emotional struggles are intertwined. I hope my book has comforted and supported you. I wish you endless days of love and light.

SHELLEY MALICOTE STUTCHMAN

NOTES AND THOUGHTS

CHAPTER FORTY-FOUR

MAN TO MAN

Cancer Post #124: Neil Talks to the Guys: May 2nd

In January, Shelley and I settled into our dream house. It was a sight to behold - the walls freshly painted, everything brand new. This home symbolized all the memories we hoped to make in our golden years together. I can still hear Shelley's voice asking me to pop open a bottle of champagne, saying it was to celebrate our new home. As we raised our glasses, joy, and contentment filled us both. Despite our ages - seventy-one for me and sixty-seven for her - we felt youthful in each other's company. When I looked at her, she was more beautiful than ever before, radiating positivity and vitality. Her optimistic outlook on life was like a breath of fresh air.

Excitement beamed across our faces as we explored our new home and discussed ideas for decorating it. I reassured her that she had free reign to transform the house in any way she pleased. Her grin was a sight to behold.

Shelley and I had big plans for February—a trip to Vegas. I wanted to see the extravagant Year of the Tiger display at the Bellagio, and we both needed some relaxation after the move and before our June wedding.

But as we roamed around the city, I couldn't help but notice she seemed more tired than usual. Don't get me wrong, she was still having a great time, but that spark that always lights up her eyes was duller. I figured it was all the stress from moving and the upcoming wedding.

I looked at Shelley sitting by my side at the bar. It was the break of dawn, and we were sipping our go-to coffee, the Nutty Irishman. Seeing her enjoying video poker made me feel happy, thinking that the golden years of our lives had arrived and would be good.

Upon our return from Vegas, we were met with a three-day delay due to ice storms in Oklahoma. We finally arrived at our new house, relieved to be settled, but I noticed a change in Shelley's demeanor. Her usual energy seemed drained, and she barely moved after work, only mustering the strength to join me for dinner when called. I worried about her - perhaps working full-time at sixty-seven was taking its toll? Or maybe the move had been too strenuous for her? But deep down, I couldn't shake the feeling that something else might be going on.

I wracked my brain, searching for a way to make retirement feasible for her. The future loomed ahead of us, waiting to be explored. I wanted the simple pleasure of lazy mornings spent with Shelley, sipping coffee and enjoying each other's company without any worries about money or work.

PEEK-A-BOOB

It was time for Shelley's yearly mammogram. We both knew there was no reason to be concerned, so she went alone as usual. She was diligent with her monthly self-exams and never felt anything unusual.

The X-rays revealed an abnormality, and the testing center's office manager set a time for further testing. I accompanied her to every appointment, putting on a brave face to hide my own worry. Deep down, I hoped it was just a harmless growth or cyst. Despite her anxieties, I reassured her there was no need to jump to conclusions. It was most likely a benign issue that could easily be addressed.

After the biopsy, we went back to see the doctor. The doctor's official words echoed in my mind, clinical and cold. "Breast cancer" – two words that had barged into our existence, uninvited and unwelcome. They threatened to unravel everything we held dear.

As the reality of Shelley's diagnosis settled over me, I allowed myself a moment to grieve for the normalcy we had just lost. My heart was heavy with the thought of what was to come: the grueling treatments and the unpredictable outcomes.

Shelley had always been the strongest person I knew. She never let any obstacle defeat her, and I was in awe of her resilience during our courtship. But now, it was my turn to be her rock. As we faced the daunting challenge of breast cancer together, I promised to do everything in my power to protect her and ease her burden.

My determination to see her through this battle grew stronger each day, fueled by my desire to shield her from harm. I made a vow: I would stand by her side every step of the way, no matter how difficult the journey may be. We were a team; she would not have to fight this alone.

I sensed her constant need for reassurance and knew she was battling her inner turmoil. Every day, I promised her we would conquer this as a team.

I was afraid, but didn't feel I could let Shelley know. After all, she was the one facing all the cancer surgeries and treatments. The words, breast cancer, seemed so foreign to me. At first, it was hard to say those two words out loud because it made everything too real. But they were real, and their potency was undeniable. I grappled in my mind with the magnitude of what lay ahead.

The doctor outlined the plan: surgery, followed by radiation or chemo, depending on the analysis of the tumor. I'd grab Shelley's hand during all the appointments following the diagnosis. I told myself I was there to support her, but honestly, it was just as much for my own sanity.

My thoughts waged a war, consumed by an unknown future. Would our dreams of travel and adventure ever come to fruition? Could we still find joy amidst the turmoil she faced every day? Guilt gnawed at me as I questioned my own concerns.

I remember grasping every word her medical team spoke about success rates. Being logical, I always prepared for the worst and hoped for the best.

Although Shelley tried to remain strong, I saw the pain in her eyes. Every tear she shed felt like a stab to my own heart. It was one of the most challenging times of my life to see her suffer like this.

I was a retired CFO, always wanting to stay ahead of the game and have a plan. But this unknown future kept me up at night, my mind racing with possibilities and worries. "We'll take it one day at a time," I reassured Shelley, repeating it like a mantra. Maybe she needed to hear it, or perhaps it was just as much for my comfort. We talked a lot about her fears and hopes, but I didn't communicate mine much. I didn't want to burden her with anything more. So many nights when the house was still, it was a stark contrast to the chaos swirling inside me.

I experienced a spiritual battle with God. Shelley, my life partner, who it took me almost seventy years to find, was diagnosed with breast cancer. How could God let such a thing happen to someone so full of life? I had many a night I asked God, "Why?"

I never got an answer. So, I read everything I could, searching for the reason. I wish I could say I found the answer, but I didn't.

I felt the weight of her cancer financially. Shelley contributed significantly to our combined income. It was my responsibility to figure out how to make it all work. I wanted to do everything I could so she didn't have to worry about missing work to get well. I spent a lot of time on what-if thoughts and what stocks I could sell if needed. However, I was grateful we had stocks. We weren't planning on dipping into them so soon after all the expenses we had recently incurred with the house. Our savings for nice dinners were now redirected to cold clinics and sterile rooms. As her husband-to-be and confidant, I knew what must be done. In this battle, one we never anticipated nor wished for, I had to make sound financial judgments.

Shelley had an overwhelming number of decisions to make. What were the potential risks and side effects of each option? How long would it take for her to recover? Should she explore alternative treatments? As men, our instinct is to tell our partners what we think they should do. But in this situation, we need to listen and support them while they make these tough choices. We can offer to help with research and provide resources, but ultimately, the decisions are theirs. And the last thing we want is to give them bad advice at such a critical time. Just be there for your partner, regardless of their chosen path.

We both appreciated our friends' generosity and willingness to help. But Shelley had an unexpected reaction - she didn't want them around during her recovery. Shelley confided in me that she felt like she would have to entertain them and simply didn't have the energy for it. So, I took on the task of expressing our gratitude, sparing her from any further stress or obligation.

For us, ritual became a source of solace. We'd sit together sipping coffee in the mornings and watch the hummingbirds flutter to their feeders in the evening. Mundane routines became cherished moments in our uncertain world. And I realized it's not about being fearless but finding the bravery to confront our fears hand in hand.

I'll always remember the day of her surgery. I was terrified for both of us. The mind plays cruel tricks, making me think she might not make it through the surgery. I didn't want to live without her. But before they wheeled her away, in front of those strangers in scrubs, I gave her a kiss and told her I loved her. It wasn't easy for me to show emotion like that in front of people I didn't know. But for Shelley, I knew I had to step out of my comfort zone. As I waited for her to come back, all I could hear was the soft hum of machines. It felt like there was nothing left inside me, with her lying on that operating table and me stuck in the waiting room. All I could think was how she shouldn't have to go through this. "Through sickness and health," I thought to myself. It wasn't a promise we made at the altar, not yet anyway, but it held just as much weight, just as much sacredness and truth.

As soon as we got home, I studied the instructions the doctor had given me. Taking care of her wounds made me anxious, but it turned out to be simple, and my worries were unfounded. The painkillers kept her comfortable for the first few days. While she rested, I stayed close by, tending to her needs and making sure she was well taken care of. She slept most of the time when I checked on her, but as long as she wasn't in pain, that was all that mattered. Remember, after surgery, your partner is suffering both physically and emotionally. Don't expect her to express gratitude for your efforts - just do what needs to be done to ease her discomfort, and don't feel unacknowledged. That's what being a good partner is all about.

A week had passed, and she was back to her usual routine of sipping coffee with me in the mornings. But something seemed off. I could tell there was a weight on her mind, and I didn't want to push her to talk about it. Eventually, she opened up to me. Women tend to talk things out, you know? A few days later, she turned off Netflix and sat me down in the living room. I could sense that this was going to be serious. She bravely told me if I didn't want to go through with the wedding because of her breast cancer, she would understand. It wasn't what we signed up for when we got engaged. It was a selfless act from her, driven by love and fear of burdening me with the uncertain road ahead.

Without hesitation, I looked at her and said, "Let's get married today."

I saw a big smile on her face, and she said, "Good answer."

She told me by my proposal to get married now, she finally realized I wasn't scared of facing the uncertain future with her and whatever mangled mess was under the wrappings around her chest. She wanted to wait until our scheduled date when all our loved ones could be present.

I realized love wasn't about some idealized body. It was about being there for someone who means everything to you, no matter the obstacles. I made a vow to myself right then and there that she wouldn't face a single day of this battle alone. We had a long road ahead with treatments before the big day, but planning for our future together gave her hope and distraction from the cancer. My advice for you? Find something meaningful that you two can look forward to in the future. Maybe it's not a wedding, but a trip to that place she's always dreamed of visiting. Keep her focused on what lies ahead for you both.

The day finally came for her dressings and corset to be removed. She was nervous because she told me to be prepared; she might look like Frankenstein. Before we began unwrapping the gauze, I told her I wasn't a boob man anyway. I liked the girl next door look, and she had that look. We were both surprised that her left breast was still intact. It was just scarred up and hollow-looking on one side. No matter what lies under all the wrappings and dressings of your partner, this is the time to be super supportive of her and put your own thoughts aside. And who cares about boobs anyway? Your partner is alive, and cancer isn't inside of her anymore.

The next step was radiation therapy. The radiologist explained the different radiation options for her breast cancer treatment. Shelley was drawn to Brachytherapy because it could all be done in one week, twice a day. The doctor assured us it wouldn't hurt too much, even though she'd have 18 tubes going in and out of her breast, making a total of 36 holes. My wife mentioned our upcoming wedding in June, and the doctor said Shelley needed to heal from the partial mastectomy and lymph node removal first. She would schedule the radiation for early May. We were both satisfied with that plan.

When we got home Shelley asked me to start wearing my wedding band, even though we weren't married yet. She said it gave her a sense of security. It took me some time to understand that her constant need for security stemmed from her own insecurities. I was already doing everything I could to make her feel loved and secure. But remember, guys - don't let your frustrations get the best of you when it comes to your partner's emotional needs. Take a deep breath and remember to always show understanding and compassion and smile.

She went back to work and got involved in a breast cancer group called P-31. They had this class at our church called Staring Cancer in the Faith, and she wanted me to go with her. I know, I know, hanging out in a room full of women talking about their breast issues was not exactly my idea of a good time. But Shelley wanted me there, and I couldn't let her down. So, there I was, the only guy in a room full of women talking about breast stuff. Kinda awkward, but I stuck it out. After the first class, I asked the leader if I should drop out. I didn't want to make the ladies uncomfortable. She assured me that I was welcome to stay. In the second session, Shelley poured her heart out about how she couldn't understand why this happened to her at the best time of her life. It must have scared off a few women because Shelley wasn't just blindly praising God and leaning on him like they seemed to be doing. Those women didn't come back for the next session. But I kept going and promised her I would see it through. Even if they were controversial, Shelley never hesitated to tackle the tough issues. Sometimes, it made me cringe inside, but I was proud of her for having the courage to ask the hard questions.

The P-31 group turned out to be a lifesaver for Shelley. One night, her arm started throbbing with pain, and a lump appeared in her elbow. We were terrified, thinking the cancer had returned. But then she reached out to the P-31 Facebook page, and within minutes, a woman gave us an answer - lymphedema. She provided a hotline for more information. Even at eleven o'clock at night, the nurse who called us back reassured us that it wasn't cancer and suggested Shelley speak to her oncologist about seeing a lymphatic massage therapist. Shelley made the appointment and was given a compression sleeve to wear along with therapy sessions. I'll be honest; convincing her, she looked fine with the sleeve was no easy feat. Don't think the battle is over after the primary surgery. From my experience, it was just the beginning. I'm sharing this with you so you can be prepared that your partner's breast cancer is an ongoing fight even after the surgery. Guys, if she doesn't take the initiative on her own to join a breast cancer support group, I encourage you to find what's available in your area and talk to her about it.

We got the clear to have sex again. I was afraid of touching Shelley's breast. I didn't want to cause her pain. Our job as husbands or partners is to make our partner feel beautiful and learn to touch her without hurting her. Yeah, it's not as easy as it used to be, but that doesn't mean it can't be intimate and fulfilling. Being an older guy had its advantages - sex is more about connecting than just having fun. But for you young guys out there, I understand it would be difficult. Suppose your partner has estrogen-positive cancer and is on hormone blockers. In that case, her libido will be lower, and she could be struggling with body image issues. Don't let this create distance in your relationship. Seek help from a sex therapist if needed. Keep the love alive, and don't let cancer win in the bedroom.

Can you believe it? The doctors pushed back Shelley's Brachytherapy until June 6th. Our wedding was to be held on June 17th, for crying out loud! Shelley begged and pleaded, but they wouldn't budge because of their precious vacations. I mean, how could they do this to us? How was Shelley supposed to recover in just six days before our big day? I was fuming at those inconsiderate doctors, but I knew I had to keep my cool for Shelley's sake. It took all my willpower not to march down to that radiology department and give them a piece of my mind. But I knew that would upset Shelley even more. Sometimes, you just want to fight the system for your woman, but you have to think about what she would want you to do. Counting to ten helps.

As weeks passed, the dust settled, and life slowly returned to a new normal. Shelley resumed her job. We didn't mention the C-word as frequently, but just when we thought we were in the clear... BAM! It was time for her radiation treatments. I saw the fear in her eyes as doctors inserted these long tubes into her left breast, with thirty-six holes, no less. She looked like some kind of twisted science experiment. I couldn't even begin to imagine what she was going through. All I could think was there had to be better ways to fight cancer that wasn't so brutal.

I'll never forget the feeling of triumph as we rang that bell together on June 10th. And let me tell you, buddy, don't skip a celebration like that. You take her out for a fancy dinner and make it a tradition to celebrate each month of being cancer-free. It's a powerful bond between partners, celebrating life and conquering that beast every month. Trust me, it's pretty cool.

Shelley was a warrior on our wedding day. Her left side was swollen from the treatment, and she didn't have much energy, but she still skipped down the aisle with her sister. Yes, the two of them skipped. When I saw her skipping towards me as my future wife, my heart couldn't help but skip a beat. Our wedding was pure hippie vibes - a short ceremony, lots of food, an open bar, and non-stop dancing. Despite everything we had been through, we had the time of our lives, as did our guests. But, when it was just Shelley and me in our honeymoon suite that night, she was utterly wiped out, and I was, too. We didn't consummate our marriage on our wedding night. But sometimes, your partner's health comes before sex, and that's just how it is. We left for our honeymoon a couple of days later, and the loving sex we had was gentle and slow. And yeah, I wondered if our wild and spontaneous sex days were over. However, as long as I have my wife by my side for years to come, who cares about all that other stuff?

After our honeymoon, my wife started on inhibitors to lower her chances of recurrence. But the side effects were brutal - she was like a frail old lady in just four months. Her body ached, she gained weight, and she was all over the place emotionally. But the worst part? She was losing her sharp mind. She came to me for advice on whether to quit the medication or not. And I'll admit, it's tough not to want to take control of the situation and tell her what's best. But we have to remember that it's ultimately her decision. My wife decided that quality of life was more important than quantity. And guess what? Just two weeks off the drug, and she was back to her usual self - no more foggy brain and stiff joints. So, trust me when I say be patient and let your woman call the shots when it comes to her cancer treatment. No matter how long you've been together, you're not a mind reader and can't dictate her choices. Support and listen instead of trying to fix things for her. She knows what's best for herself.

You might think my recount would end here, but no. The Susan B. Komen organization nominated me as a Pink Tie Guy. Yes, it was an honor. You're being recognized for supporting your loved one through their breast cancer journey. You have to do some fundraising and attend a fancy banquet. I was proud to be nominated, but I'm not a center-stage guy. I didn't want to get up in front of a large crowd of people, have something read about me, and accept my award. Plus, I'm a Hawaiian shirt, shorts, and tennis shoes kind of man. I hated wearing suits, which I would have to wear. However, Shelley was head over heels thrilled when she learned about my award. I told her I wasn't comfortable accepting the nomination and being the center of attention. Then she gave me that look and a slight pout, so I accepted. Here's my advice: don't be afraid to step out of your comfort zone for the ones you love. You only know how much it means to them once you do it. Be that Pink Tie Guy with pride because your loved one deserves it.

As time moved forward in our life together, we learned that love isn't about what you can do for each other but rather what you can do together. This unbreakable bond is a testament to your commitment and love's power and ability to conquer even the toughest of challenges.

The End and The Beginning

SHELLEY MALICOTE STUTCHMAN

NOTES AND THOUGHTS

Acknowledgements

Creative Quills (Our Leader Andrea Foster and all my CQAuthor Friends)

P31 Breast Cancer Support Group

My Livestrong Tribe

BreastCancer Fighters & Survivors of Oklahoma

Book Cover Models and Survivors: Sally Cable, Jackie Damiani, Jodi Cooper, Lynette Green, Loreen Moore, Willow LaMunyon, TerJuana Brooks

Epworth Villa Staff and Residents

Epworth at Home Team

All my family, friends, Facebook and TikTok friends, and medical team.

About the author

SHELLEY MALICOTE STUTCHMAN, SURVIVOR

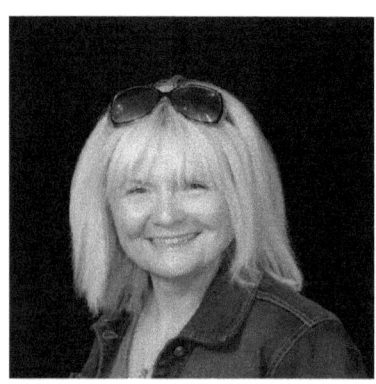
Shelley Stutchman has triumphed over breast cancer and emerged as a dedicated patient advocate. Her journey as a retired nurse and former community liaison for home health and hospice has endowed her with invaluable firsthand experience in the medical field. Her passion for research is not just a mere sentiment but a commitment she demonstrated by becoming a test subject for Moderna's COVID-19 vaccine.

Shelley has owned a mental health program for low-income women, founded a support group for women over forty, and received recognition from the governor for her work with Workforce Oklahoma.

She also excels in public speaking, winning multiple awards through Toastmasters International. Shelley is a featured writer for CAREGIVER MAGAZINE and has won awards in writing contests.

Shelley's love for writing and storytelling is a testament to her creative spirit. She inherited this passion from her great uncle, Maurice Kelley, a renowned author and English professor at Princeton University. Today, she shares her own stories through various platforms, including creating daily videos on TikTok and being a Facebook Digital Creator.

When she's not writing or advocating, Shelley enjoys life's simple pleasures—like watching hummingbirds on her front porch with her husband Neil Johnson, aka Cameraman.

Shelley offers speaking engagements on breast cancer to spread awareness and inspire others to keep fighting.

Thank you

Thank you so much for taking the time to read my book. I hope it has been informative and helpful in understanding breast cancer. I urge you to dig deeper and expand your knowledge on this topic. Remember, knowledge is power in the fight against breast cancer.

For inquiries about speaking engagements, please contact me at Medicarejetsetters@gmail.com.

Thank you again for your support.

Love & Peace,

Shelley Malicote Stutchman

Unveiling the Soul of Quotes

I love quotes and am constantly looking for new ones that can bring me joy, motivation, inspiration, or simply make me smile. I hope that the quotes I have compiled in this book will bring you the same sense of comfort and empowerment that they have brought me.

(Page 8) "Half the worry in the world is caused by people trying to make decisions before they have sufficient knowledge on which to base a decision."
—Herbert E. Hawkes

(Page 12) "Trust yourself. You've survived a lot, and you'll survive whatever is coming."
—Robert Tew

(Page 16) "When you get diagnosed with cancer, there's such a sense of loneliness, but what we need to know as people going through this is that you're not alone."
—Christina Applegate

(Page 21) "If it takes a village to raise a child, it takes a bloody army to battle cancer."
—Niyati Tamaskar

(Page 26) "Once I overcame breast cancer, I wasn't afraid of anything anymore."
—Melissa Etheridge

(Page 28) "Every woman needs to know the facts. And the fact is, when it comes to breast cancer, every woman is at risk."
—Debbie Wasserman Schultz

(Page 30) "The period of greatest gain in knowledge and experience is the most difficult period in one's life."
—Dalai Lama

(Page 33) "Breathe, darling; this is just a chapter and not the end."
—S.C. Lourie

(Page 36) "Breast cancer is scary and no one understands that like another woman who has gone through it too."
—Mindy Sterling

(Page 38) "It's our challenges and obstacles that give us layers of depth and make us interesting. Are they fun when they happen? No. But they are what make us unique. And that's what I know for sure… I think."
—Ellen Degeneres

(Page 43) "Always remember that your present situation is not your final destination. The best is yet to come." —Anonymous

(Page 45) "With the new day comes new strength and new thoughts."
—Eleanor Roosevelt

(Page 51) "God, Winks are better than coffee and chocolate!"
—Shelley Stutchman

(Page 55) "We have two options, medically and emotionally: give up or fight like hell."
—Lance Armstrong

(Page 57) "Do not partner with fear to help you make decisions."
—Jeannette Gregory

(Page 64) "Before I started chemotherapy treatments, I wrote down the best advice from doctors, family, friends, books, and survivors and created an 'Owner's Manual' to help me take care of myself. It would remind me that cancer is doable."
—Regina Brett

(Page 68) "Cancer may have started the fight, but I will finish it."
—Unknown

(Page 71) "When you have exhausted all possibilities, remember this: You haven't."
—Thomas Edison

(Page 73) "For beautiful eyes, look for the good in others; for beautiful lips, speak only words of kindness; and for poise, walk with the knowledge that you are never alone."
—Audrey Hepburn

(Page 74) "I'm here today because I refused to be unhappy. I took a chance."
—Wanda Sykes

(Page 77) "Keeping your body healthy is an expression of gratitude to the whole cosmos — the trees, the clouds, everything."
—Thích Nhất Hạnh

(Page 81) "I don't think of all the misery but of the beauty that still remains."
—Anne Frank

(Page 84) "More than 10 million Americans are living with cancer, and they demonstrate the ever-increasing possibility of living beyond cancer."
—Sheryl Crow

(Page 87) "Take time to be thankful for today, for tomorrow is never a guarantee."
—Shelley Stutchman

(Page 90) "When we long for life without difficulties, remind us that oaks grow strong in contrary winds, and diamonds are made under pressure."
—Peter Marshall

(Page 95) "Wine a little and you'll feel better."
—Anonymous

(Page 97) "Once you choose hope, anything's possible."
—Christopher Reeve

(Page 99) "Every negative belief weakens the partnership between mind and body."
—Deepak Chopra

(Page 101) "This poo shall pass."
—Anonymous

(Page 104) "Values are related to our emotions, just as we practice physical hygiene to preserve our physical health, we need to observe emotional hygiene to preserve a healthy mind and attitudes."
—Dalai Lama

(Page 106) "Don't be afraid to ask for help; seeking financial advice is a sign of strength, not weakness."
—Anonymous

(Page 109) "In three words I can sum up everything I've learned about life: It goes on."
—Robert Frost

(Page 111) "When in doubt take a bath."
—Mae West

(Page 113) "Self-care is not selfish. You cannot serve from an empty vessel."
—Eleanor Brownn, author

(Page 115) "Never be ashamed of a scar. It simply means you were stronger than whatever tried to hurt you."
—Unknown

(Page 119) "Health is like money; we never have a true idea of its value until we lose it.
—Josh Billings, humor writer

(Page 121) "You have to be willing to give up the life you planned, and instead, greet the life that is waiting for you."
—Joseph Campbell

(Page 125) "Hope is the ability to hear the music of the future. Faith is the courage to dance to it today."
—Peter Kuzmic

(Page 126) "Cancer changes your life, often for the better. You learn what's important, you learn to prioritize, and you learn not to waste your time. You tell people you love them."
—Joel Siegel

(Page 131) "The more you lose yourself in something bigger than yourself, the more energy you will have."
—Norman Vincent Peale

(Page 133) "Each day comes bearing its own gifts. Untie the ribbons."
—Ruth Ann Schabacker

(Page 135) "Being deeply loved by someone gives you strength, while loving someone deeply gives you courage."
—Lao Tzu

(Page 137) "A sure sign of a man's strength is how gently he loves his wife."
—FierceMarriage.com

(Page 141) "Whether you're a mother or father, or a husband or a son, or a niece or a nephew or uncle, breast cancer doesn't discriminate."
—Stephanie McMahon

(Page 145) "Toughness is in the soul and spirit, not in muscles."
—Alex Karras

(Page 150) "I am not this hair, I am not this skin, I am the soul that lives within."
—Rumi

(Page 154) "Cancer is a word, not a sentence."
—John Diamond

(Page 157) "Hope is like the sun, which, as we journey toward it, casts the shadow of our burden behind us."
—Samuel Smiles

(Page 159) "Fear defeats more people than any other thing in the world."
—Ralph Waldo Emerson

(Page 164) "A generation ago breast cancer was a dreaded disease spoken about in hushed tones by our mothers...The survival rate was only 50% and mastectomy was inevitable. The story couldn't be more different today. Survival rates are soaring and treatment by lumpectomy or with reconstruction means avoiding disfigurement....I believe that breast cancer will soon become something we live with rather than die from."
—Lindsay Nicholson, Good Housekeeping Editor and Breast Cancer Survivor

(Page 166) "How many cancer patients does it take to screw in a light bulb? Just one, but they have a big support group cheering them on. We're all here for you!"
—Anonymous

(Page 169) "No matter what happens, or how bad it seems today, life does go on, and it will be better tomorrow." —Maya Angelou

(Page 173) "My cancer scare changed my life. I'm grateful for every new, healthy day I have. It has helped me prioritize my life."
—Olivia Newton-John

(Page 177) "Love and laughter are two of the most important universal cancer treatments on the planet. Overdose on them."
—Tanya Masse

(Page 181) "Life wants you to fight it. Learn how to make it your own. It wants you to grab and axe and hack through the wood. It wants you to get a sledgehammer and break through concrete. It wants you to grab a torch and burn through the metal and steel until you can reach through and grab it. Life wants you to grab all the organized, the alphabetized, the chronological, the sequenced. It wants you to mix it all together, stir it up, blend it."

—Colleen Hoover

(Page 184) "Laughter boosts the immune system and helps the body fight off disease, cancer cells as well as viral, bacterial and other infections. Being happy is the best cure of all diseases!"

—Patch Adams

(Page 186) "Cancer recovery is hard work. Life is hard work. And it really pays off. Hang in there." —Helen Szablya

(Page 188) Want to hear a terrible joke? Okay, here we go.
"Did you hear about the bee who had a tumor? Don't worry - it was BEE-nign."
—Anonymous

(Page 192) "Today will never come again. Be a blessing. Be a friend. Encourage someone. Take time to care. Let your words heal and not wound."

—Unknown

(Page 196) "God didn't promise days without pain, laughter without sorrow, or sun without rain, but He did promise strength for the day, comfort for the tears, and light for the way."

—Unknown

(Page 202) "People with a strong willpower will always have the bigger picture in mind. They will be able to forgo small pleasures in order to help attain bigger goals."

—Bryan Adams

(Page 206) "The patient's medical history has been remarkably insignificant, with only a 40-pound weight gain in the last three days."

—Unknown

(Page 208) 1. Your alarm clock goes off at 6 a.m., and you're glad to hear it.
2. Your mother-in-law invites you to lunch, and you say NO.
3. You're back in the family rotation to take out the garbage.
4. When you no longer have an urge to choke the person who says, "all you need to beat cancer is the right attitude."
5. When your dental floss runs out, and you buy 1000 yards.
6. When you use your toothbrush to brush your teeth and not comb your hair.
7. You have a chance to buy additional life insurance, but you buy a new convertible car instead.

8. Your doctor tells you to lose weight and do something about your cholesterol, and you listen.
9. When your biggest annual celebration is again your birthday and not the day you were diagnosed.
10. When you use your Visa card more than your hospital parking pass.
—Anonymous

(Page 210) "If you set goals and go after them with all the determination you can muster, your gifts will take you places that amaze you."

—Les Brown

(Page 212) "The mind, in addition to medicine, has powers to turn the immune system around."
—Jonas Salk

(Page 214) "Believe you can, and you are halfway there."
—Theodore Roosevelt

(Page 218) "It's about focusing on the fight and not the fright."
—Robin Roberts

(Page 220) "If I quit now, I will be back to where I started, & when I started, I was desperately wishing to be where I am now."
—Anonymous

(Page 222) "You didn't make it through surgery, radiation, and or chemo just to end up on the couch. Get an exercise program and get moving!"
—Unknown

(Page 226) "I think a hero is any person really intent on making this a better place for all people."
—Maya Angelou

(Page 231) "Cancer is not a death sentence, but rather it is a life sentence; it pushes one to live."
—Marcia Smith

(Page 235) "I had uterine cancer, which is the most under-funded and under-researched of all the female cancer." —Fran Drescher

(Page 238) "You are not defined by your test results. You are so much more than that."
—Unknown

(Page 240) "It is not so much our friends' help that helps us as the confident knowledge that they will help us."
—Epicurus

(Page 242) "The ultimate test of faith is not how loudly you praise God in happy times but how deeply you trust him in dark times."
—Rick Warren

(Page 244) "Anxiety is a lot like a toddler. It never stops talking, tells you you're wrong about everything, and wakes you up at 3 a.m."
—Anonymous

(Page 246) "Don't dig your grave with your own knife and fork."
—Author Unknown

(Page 248) "You don't have the power to make rainbows or waterfalls, sunsets or roses, but you do have the power to bless people by your words and smiles You carry within you the power to make the world better."
—Sharon G. Larsen

(Page 251) "The two words 'information' and 'communication' are often used interchangeably, but they signify quite different things. Information is giving out; communication is getting through."
—Sydney J. Harris

(Page 253) "Being assertive does not mean attacking or ignoring other's feelings. It means that you are willing to hold up for yourself fairly-without attacking others."
—Albert Ellis

(Page 257) "Okay, let's see if I got this straight. The butt is the new breast, and the lower back is the new ankle. Now if only we could figure out where the brain has moved."
—Celia Rivenbark

(Page 259) "The decision to be an organ donor is the embodiment of faith in the power of humanity to heal, to save and to prevail."
—Unknown

(Page 263) "Medicine is a science of uncertainty and an art of probability."
—William Osler

(Page 265) "Learning is the beginning of wealth. Learning is the beginning of health. Learning is the beginning of spirituality. Searching and learning is where the miracle process all begins."
—Jim Rohn

(Page 267) "I always say, 'Do you have a body? Then you're swimsuit ready.' That's all you need to worry about."
—Emily Ratajkowski

(Page 271) "Friends can help each other. A true friend is someone who lets you have total freedom to be yourself – and especially to feel. Or not feel. Whatever you happen to be feeling at the moment is fine with them. That's what real love amounts to – letting a person be what he really is."
—Jim Morrison

(Page 276) "Here's to the crazy ones. The misfits. The rebels. The troublemakers. The round pegs in the square holes. The ones who see things differently. They're not fond of rules. And they have no respect for the status quo. You can quote them, disagree with them, glorify or vilify them. About the only thing you can't do is ignore them. Because they change things. They push the human race forward. And while some may see them as the crazy ones, we see genius. Because the people who are crazy enough to think they can change the world, are the ones who do."
—Rob Siltanen

(Page 279) "Knowledge is the life of the mind."
—Abu Bakr As-Siddiq (RA)

(Page 281) "What is your skin trying to tell you? Often the skin is a metaphor for deeper issues and a way for your body to send up a red flag to warn you that all is not well underneath."
—Dr. Judyth Reichenberg

(Page 284) "Plenty of people will think you're crazy, no matter what you do. Don't let that stop you from finding the people who think you're incredible - the ones who need to hear your voice because it reminds them of their own. Your tribe. They're out there. Don't let your critics interfere with your search for them."
—Vironika Tugaleva

(Page 287) "Do not reward yourself with food. You are not a dog."
—Unknown

(Page 291) "Through strength, I will mend."
—Anonymous

(Page 292) "Try calling someone just to tell them you can't talk right now."
—Anonymous

(Page 295) "If he only wants you for your breasts, legs, and thighs, send him to KFC."
—Drake

(Page 297) "When life kicks you, let it kick you forward."
—Kay Yow

(Page 298) "I'm not gaining weight; I'm retaining awesomeness."
—Unknown

(Page 301) "I believe one can live many lives through personal style. Every day is an occasion to reinvent yourself."
—Ralph Lauren

(Page 303) "Genetic code is a divine writing."
—Toba Beta

(Page 305) "I saw a woman wearing a sweatshirt with 'Guess' on it So, I said, "Implants?"
—Unknown

(Page 307) "Bras are often booby-trapped."
—Tiffany Reisz

(Page 311) "Dammit I fell asleep during a Hallmark movie so now I'll never know if the cute couple who misunderstood each other at first fell in love."
—Kim Bongiorno

(Page 318) "If man made it, don't eat it."
—Jack LaLanne

(Page 321) "If you woke up this morning with more health than illness, you are more fortunate than the million people on the planet who will not survive this week. If you can attend a religious meeting without fear of harassment, arrest, torture, or death, you are more blessed than three billion people in the world."
—Ted Zeff

(Page 325) "For every minute you are angry, you lose sixty seconds of happiness."
—Ralph Waldo Emerson

(Page 328) "Give me six hours to chop down a tree and I will spend the first four sharpening the axe."
—Abraham Lincoln

(Page 332) "Turn down the volume of your negative inner voice and create a nurturing inner voice to take its place. When you make a mistake, forgive yourself, learn from it, and move on instead of obsessing about it. Equally important, don't allow anyone else to dwell on your mistakes or shortcomings or to expect perfection from you."
—Beverly Engel

(Page 336) " My cancer scare changed my life. I'm grateful for every new, healthy day I have. It has helped me prioritize my life. "

—Olivia Newton-John

(Page 338) "Jobs fill your pocket, but adventures fill your soul."

—Jamie Lyn Beatty

(Page 340) "Never bet with anyone you meet on the first tee who has a deep suntan, a 1-iron in his bag, and squinty eyes."

—Dave Marr

(Page 342) "Don't work out because you hate your body — work out because you love it."

—Unknown

(Page 344) "A bath, a candle, music, and being left alone to soak…. ah."

—Shelley Malicote Stutchman

(Page 346) "And I said to my body, softly, 'I want to be your friend.' It took a long breath. And replied, 'I have been waiting my whole life for this."

—Nayyirah Waheed

(Page 352) "Lots of people want to ride with you in the limo, but what you want is someone who will take the bus with you when the limo breaks down."

—Oprah Winfrey

(Page 357) "God gave us the gift of life; it is up to us to give ourselves the gift of living well." —Voltaire

(Page 359) "Giving in to the darkness offers no benefit."

—Marivel Preciado

(Page 363) "The most important aim of cancer treatment is to achieve cure and secondly life prolongation and relief of sufferings. We must understand the mechanisms of how cancer develops and progresses to unlock new ways to prevent, detect and treat it."

—Dr. Dinesh Kacha – Researcher

(Page 365) "If I had to choose between loving my child and breathing, I would use my last breath to tell you I love you."

—Unknown

(Page 370) "Rock on, Rockstar."
—Joel Sebring

(Page 374) "Overcoming cancer awakens a courage and confidence inside of you that makes you want to live big, bold and intentional every day. It becomes much easier to grow as a person, because you have already been forced way out of your comfort zone. I don't worry about failing when I try new things now, because my inner voice always reminds me that 'this' can't be any harder than cancer!"
—Renee Ward

(Page 379) "Here's to you—I hope that you get steadier, stronger, and better every day."
—Unknown

(Page 384) "Sex: the thing that takes up the least amount of time and causes the most amount of trouble."
—John Barrymore

(Page 388) "An individual doesn't get cancer, a family does."
—Terry Tempest Williams

(Page 391) "Twenty years from now, you will be more disappointed by the things you didn't do than those you did. So, throw off the bowlines. Sail away from safe harbor. Catch the wind in your sails. Explore. Dream. Discover."
—Mark Twain

CITATIONS FOR QUOTES

(Page 8) Agie, J. (2023, September 19). "56+ Helpful Quotes About Worrying About The Future." Kidadl. Retrieved March 20, 2024, from https://kidadl.com/quotes/helpful-quotes-about-worrying-about-the-future

(Page 12) Robert Tew. (n.d.). Quotespedia. Retrieved March 20, 2024, from https://www.quotespedia.org/authors/r/robert-tew/trust-yourself-youve-survived-a-lot-and-youll-survive-whatever-is-coming-robert-tew/

(Page 16) Gleeson, J. (2023, September 16). Country Living. 80 "Quotes for Breast Cancer Awareness Month That Inspire and Educate." Retrieved March 20, 2024, from https://www.countryliving.com/life/inspirational-stories/a45082685/breast-cancer-awareness-quotes/

(Page 21) "Unafraid Quotes. (n.d.)." goodreads. Retrieved March 22, 2024, from "https://www.goodreads.com/work/quotes/71405657-unafraid-a-survivors-quest-for-human-connection

(Page 26 and Page 28) Osmanski, S. (2022, October 7). "Never Give Up and Always Keep the Faith—75 Quotes About Breast Cancer That Resonate." Parade. Retrieved March 22, 2024, from https://parade.com/1183333/stephanieosmanski/breast-cancer-quotes/

(Page 30) Dalai Lama Quotes About Suffering. (n.d.). AZ Quotes. Retrieved March 22, 2024, from https://www.azquotes.com/author/8418-Dalai_Lama/tag/suffering

(Page 33) World Cancer Day Quotes. (2023, February 26). 143 Greetings.com. Retrieved March 22, 2024, from https://www.143greetings.com/world-cancer-day-quotes.html

(Page 36) Wolkenhauer, A. (2023, August 25). 32 Inspiring Breast Cancer Quotes to Share with a Loved One. cake. Retrieved March 23, 2024, from https://www.joincake.com/blog/breast-cancer-awareness-quotes/

(Page 38) Ellen DeGeneres Quotes. (n.d.). Brainy Quote. Retrieved March 24, 2024, from https://www.brainyquote.com/quotes/ellen_degeneres_451764

(Page 43) Zig Ziglar > Quotes > Quotable Quote. (n.d.). goodreads. Retrieved March 24, 2024, from https://www.goodreads.com/quotes/915549-always-remember-that-your-present-situation-is-not-your-final

(Page 45) Druce, M. (2023, January 27). Breast Cancer Quotes from Breast Cancer Warriors – 100+ Inspirational Quotes. The Breslow Center. Retrieved March 25, 2024, from https://www.breslowmd.com/breast-cancer-quotes/

(Page 55) Lance Armstrong Quote. (n.d.). Lib Quotes. Retrieved March 26, 2024, from https://libquotes.com/lance-armstrong/quote/lbo4c1e

(Page 57) Osmanski, S. (2022, October 7)."Never Give Up and Always Keep the Faith—75 Quotes About Breast Cancer That Resonate." Parade. Retrieved March 26, 2024, from https://parade.com/1183333/stephanieosmanski/breast-cancer-quotes/

(Page 64) Brett, R. (n.d.). Chemotherapy Quotes. Brainy Quotes. Retrieved June 18, 2024, from https://www.brainyquote.com/quotes/regina_brett_586753?src=t_chemotherapy

(Page 68) Connealy, L. E. (2023, August 12). "Inspiring Uplifting Cancer Quotes: Strength, Courage & Hope." Cancer Center for Healing. Retrieved March 26, 2024, from https://cancercenterforhealing.com/uplifting-cancer-quotes/

(Page 71) Team of Fearless Motivation. (2018, July 4). Thomas Edison Quotes – Failure IS the Road to Success!. Fearless Motivation. Retrieved March 27, 2024, from https://www.fearlessmotivation.com/2018/07/04/thomas-edison-quotes/

(Page 73) Audrey Hepburn Quotes . (n.d.). Brainy Quote. Retrieved March 27, 2024, from https://www.brainyquote.com/quotes/audrey_hepburn_394440

(Page 74) Medrut, F. (n.d.)."25 Wanda Sykes Quotes That Are Both Funny and Inspirational. Goalcast. Retrieved March 27, 2024, from https://www.goalcast.com/wanda-sykes-quotes/

(Page 77) Lim, E. (n.d.). "15 Best Mindfulness Quotes by Thich Nhat Hanh." Evelyn Lim. Retrieved March 29, 2024, from https://www.evelynlim.com/mindfulness-quotes-thich-nhat-hanh/

(Page 81) Tscherry, L. (2015, January 27)." Anne Frank: 10 beautiful quotes from The Diary of a Young Girl." The Gaurdian. https://www.theguardian.com/childrens-books-site/2015/jan/27/the-greatest-anne-frank-quotes-ever

(Page 84) Osmanski, S. (2022, October 7). "Never Give Up and Always Keep the Faith—75 Quotes About Breast Cancer That Resonate." Parade. Retrieved March 29, 2024, from https://parade.com/1183333/stephanieosmanski/breast-cancer-quotes/

(Page 90) Peter Marshall Quotes. (n.d.). AZ Quotes. Retrieved March 30, 2024, from https://www.azquotes.com/author/9514-Peter_Marshall

(Page 95) Eventful Words. (2023, April 5). "105 Best Inspirational Wine Quotes to Lift Your Spirits."

(Page 97) Christopher Reeve Quotes. (n.d.). AZ Quotes. Retrieved April 1, 2024, from https://www.azquotes.com/author/12181-Christopher_Reeve

(Page 99) Chopra, D. (2013, November 8). "Negative Beliefs." Deepak Chopra. Retrieved April 1, 2024, from https://www.deepakchopra.com/articles/negative-beliefs/

(Page 101) (n.d.). AZ Quotes. Retrieved April 2, 2024, from https://www.azquotes.com/quote/1269767

(Page 104) Cruz, G. (2023, July 21). "101 Inspirational Quotes For Financial Problems: Overcoming With Resilience."

(Page 106) Let's Learn Slang. Retrieved April 2, 2024, from https://letslearnslang.com/inspirational-quotes-for-financial-problems/

(Page 109) In Three Words, I Can Sum Up Everything I've Learned About Life. It Goes On Posted byquoteresearch April 1, 2018 . (2018, April 1). Quote Investigator. Retrieved April 3, 2024, from https://quoteinvestigator.com/2018/04/01/life-goes/

(Page 111) West, M. (n.d.). Baths Quotes. AZ Quotes. Retrieved May 24, 2024, from https://www.azquotes.com/quote/910946?ref=baths

(Page 113) Brownn, E. (2014, November 2). SELF-CARE IN NOT SELFISH. Eleanor Brownn. Retrieved April 3, 2024, from http://www.eleanorbrownn.com/blog2/self-care-in-not-selfish

(Page 115) Browne, R. (n.d.). "How to Rock Your Scars (Because They Mean You're Strong)." tiny buddha. Retrieved April 3, 2024, from https://tinybuddha.com/blog/never-ashamed-scar-4-lessons-self-acceptance-resilience/

(Page 119) Josh Billings Quotes. (n.d.). AZ Quotes. https://www.azquotes.com/author/1398-Josh_Billings

(Page 121) Caring Bridge Staff. (2022, October 12). "20 Encouraging Cancer Quotes for Patients to Inspire Hope." Caring Bridge. Retrieved April 3, 2024, from https://www.caringbridge.org/resources/encouraging-cancer-quotes-to-inspire-hope/

(Page 125) Seedbed. (2014, February 6). 2.6.14 "Epiphany Means Hearing The Music Of The Future...." Wake-Up Call. Retrieved April 4, 2024, from https://seedbed.com/salvation-belongs-to-our-god/

(Page 126) Hopeful Quotes. (n.d.). Rogel Cancer Center. Retrieved April 4, 2024, from https://www.rogelcancercenter.org/living-with-cancer/sharing-hope/hopeful-quotes

(Page 131 The Strive. (n.d.)."50+ NORMAN VINCENT PEALE QUOTES ON THE POWER OF POSITIVE THOUGHT." The Strive. Retrieved April 4, 2024, from https://thestrive.co/norman-vincent-peale-quotes/

(Page 133) Thought for the Day: Schabacker (2018, December 30). EVERYDAY INTENTIONAL LIVING. Retrieved April 4, 2024, from https://everydayintentionalliving.com/thought-for-the-day-schabacker/

(Page 135) Lao Tzu > Quotes > Quotable Quote. (n.d.). Good Reads. Retrieved April 4, 2024, from https://www.goodreads.com/quotes/2279-being-deeply-loved-by-someone-gives-you-strength-while-loving

(Page 137) Frederick, R. (n.d.). Fierce Marriage. "CHRISTIAN MARRIAGE QUOTES." Retrieved April 4, 2024, from https://christianmarriagequotes.com/2398-a-sure-sign-of-a-mans-strength-is-how-gently-he-loves-his-wife-3/

(Page 141) Osmanski, S. (2022, October 7)."Never Give Up and Always Keep the Faith—75 Quotes About Breast Cancer That Resonate." Parade. Retrieved April 5, 2024, from https://parade.com/1183333/stephanieosmanski/breast-cancer-quotes/

(Page 145) Quotes > Authors > A > Alex Karras . (n.d.). AZ Quotes. Retrieved April 5, 2024, from https://www.azquotes.com/quote/524447

(Page 150) Featured in:" Rumi Quotes, Soul Quotes." (n.d.). Quote Fancy. Retrieved April 5, 2024, from https://quotefancy.com/quote/904147/Rumi-I-am-not-this-hair-I-am-not-this-skin-I-am-the-soul-that-lives-within

(Page 154) Featured in: John Diamond Quotes. (n.d.). Quote Fancy. Retrieved April 5, 2024, from https://quotefancy.com/quote/1584644/John-Diamond-Cancer-is-a-word-not-a-sentence#:~:text=John%20Diamond%20Quote%3A%20%E2%80%9CCancer%20is,word%2C%20not%20a%20sentence.%E2%80%9D

(Page 157) Smiles, S. (n.d.). Statustown. Retrieved April 6, 2024, from https://statustown.com/quote/34855/

(Page 159) Ralph Waldo Emerson Quotes. (n.d.). Brainy Quote. Retrieved April 6, 2024, from https://www.brainyquote.com/quotes/ralph_waldo_emerson_134898

(Page 164) Nicholson, L. (2014, September 26). https://www.goodhousekeeping.com/uk/health/health-advice/g544799/inspirational-quotes-from-breast-cancer-survivors/?slide=2. Good Housekeeping. Retrieved April 6, 2024, from https://www.goodhousekeeping.com/uk/health/health-advice/g544799/inspirational-quotes-from-breast-cancer-survivors/?slide=2

(Page 166) Workman, J. (2013, October 20). "HOW MANY CANCER PATIENTS DOES IT TAKE TO CHANGE A LIGHT BULB?" JANWORKMAN. Retrieved April 6, 2024, from https://janworkman.com/2013/10/20/how-many-cancer-patients-does-it-take-to-change-a-light-bulb/

(Page 169) Fielding, S., & Caldwell, S. (2024, April 5). "These wise quotes from Maya Angelou will inspire you every day." Today. Retrieved April 6, 2024, from https://www.yahoo.com/lifestyle/25-maya-angelous-most-iconic-020107282.html

(Pag 173) Olivia Newton-John. (n.d.). AZQuotes.com. Retrieved June 23, 2024, from AZQuotes.com Web site: https://www.azquotes.com/quote/565190

(Page 177) Tanya Masse > Quotes > Quotable Quote. (n.d.). Goodreads. Retrieved April 6, 2024, from https://www.goodreads.com/quotes/6682199-love-and-laughter-are-two-of-the-most-important-universal

(Page 181) "Slammed Quotes." (n.d.). good reads. Retrieved April 7, 2024, from https://www.goodreads.com/work/quotes/18602144-slammed

(Page 184) Patch Adam's Quotes. (n.d.). Quote Fancy. Retrieved April 7, 2024, from https://quotefancy.com/quote/1521531/Patch-Adams-Laughter-boosts-the-immune-system-and-helps-the-body-fight-off-disease-cancer

(Page 186) Vogel, K. (2020, December 23). "150 Inspiring Quotes on Beating Cancer from Super Survivors." Parade. Retrieved April 7, 2024, from https://parade.com/1140135/kaitlin-vogel/cancer-quotes/

(Page 188) Wright, K. (2020, January 1). 34 Funny & Cheerful Messages for Cancer Patients. Cake. Retrieved June 28, 2024, from https://www.joincake.com/blog/humorous-words-of-encouragement-for-cancer-patients/

(Page 192) (2024, April 8). Daily Inspirational Quotes. Retrieved April 8, 2024, from https://www.dailyinspirationalquotes.in/2015/10/today-will-never-come-again-be-a-blessing-be-a-friend-encourage-someone-take-time-to-care-let-your-words-heal-and-not-wound/

(Page 196) "115 Beautiful And Inspiring Faith Quotes And Sayings." (n.d.). ask IDEAS. Retrieved April 8, 2024, from https://www.askideas.com/top-115-beautiful-and-inspiring-faith-quotes-and-sayings/god-didnt-promise-days-without-pain-laughter-without-sorrow-or-sun-without-rain-but-he-did-promise-strength-for-the-da

(Page 202) "My top 10 quotes on Willpower." (n.d.). dorie massumi. Retrieved April 8, 2024, from https://www.dmnewplacement.ch/en/news-details/my-top-10-quotes-on-willpower-869.html

(Page 206) Murray, S. (2020, January 5). "The Best of Medical Chart Errors." HCP Line. Retrieved April 9, 2024, from https://www.hcplive.com/view/the-best-of-medical-chart-errors/1000

(Page 208) "Sometimes We Just Need Humor." (n.d.). WHOOPS. Retrieved April 9, 2024, from https://www.cancerabcs.org/cancer-humor

(Page 210) Les Brown Quote. (n.d.). Brainy Quote. https://www.brainyquote.com/quotes/les_brown_391112

(Page 212) Jonas Salk Quotes. (n.d.). Quote Fancy. Retrieved April 9, 2024, from https://quotefancy.com/quote/1398221/Jonas-Salk-The-mind-in-addition-to-medicine-has-powers-to-turn-the-immune-system-around#:~:text=Jonas%20Salk%20Quote%3A%20E2%80%9CThe%20mind,turn%20the%20immune%2

(Page 214) Mind Blood. (n.d.). "Believe you can and you're halfway there." Mind Blood. Retrieved April 9, 2024, from https://mindblood.com/believe-you-can-and-youre-halfway-there-theodore-roosevelt/

(Page 218) "Robin Roberts Quotes." (n.d.). quote fancy. Retrieved April 9, 2024, from https://quotefancy.com/quote/1386092/Robin-Roberts-It-s-about-focusing-on-the-fight-and-not-the-fright

(Page 220) "anonymous quotes." (n.d.). quote fancy. Retrieved April 10, 2024, from https://quotefancy.com /quote/2780781/Anonymous-If-I-quit-now-I-will-soon-be-back-to-where-I-started-And-when-I-started-I-was

(Page 222) "44 Inspirational Hero Quotes To Be The Best Version Of You." (n.d.). Habit Stacker. Retrieved April 12, 2024, from https://thehabitstacker.com/hero-quotes/

(Page 226) Parkerton, M. (2023, March 5). "101 Inspirational and Uplifting Quotes to Encourage Hope in Cancer Patients." Parade. Retrieved April 12, 2024, from https://parade.com/1178471/michelle-parkerton/inspirational-cancer-quotes/

(Page 231) Lowthert, J. (2014, December 30). 16 Quotes To Encourage Cancer Patients. ThoughtCatalog. Retrieved June 27, 2024, from https://thoughtcatalog.com/jenna-lowthert/2014/12/16-quotes-to-encourage-cancer-patients/

(Page 235) "Fran Drescher Quotes." (n.d.). quotefancy. Retrieved April 14, 2024, from https://quotefancy.com/quote/1167383/Fran-Drescher-I-had-uterine-cancer-which-is-the-most-under-funded-and-under-researched-of

(Page 238) Tag Vault. (2023, April 23). "107+ Words of Encouragement for Someone Waiting for Test Results" [Medical, Academic]. Tag Vault. Retrieved April 14, 2024, from https://tagvault.org/blog/words-of-encouragement-someone-waiting-test-results/

(Page 240) "Epicurus Quotes." (n.d.). quote fancy. Retrieved April 15, 2024, from https://quotefancy.com /quote/55214/Epicurus-It-is-not-so-much-our-friends-help-that-helps-us-as-the-confident-knowledge-that

(Page 242) "Rick Warren Quotes." (n.d.). quote fancy. Retrieved April 15, 2024, from https://quotefancy.com/quote/899414/Rick-Warren-The-ultimate-test-of-faith-is-not-how-loudly-you-praise-God-in-happy-times

(Page 244) Stiles, K. (2021, July 30). 45 Quotes About Anxiety. Psych Central. Retrieved April 15, 2024, from https://psychcentral.com/anxiety/quotes-about-anxiety

(Page 246) Don't Dig Your Grace with Your Own Fork and Knife (2024, June 27). Once in a Blue Moon. Retrieved June 27, 2024, from https://onceinabluemoon.ca/dont-dig-your-grave-with-your-own-knife-and-fork/

(Page 248) "Blessing To Others Quotes." (n.d.). AZ Quotes. Retrieved April 15, 2024, from https://www.azquotes.com/quotes/topics/blessing-to-others.html

(Page: 251): Schulmeister, L. (2017, December 21). "Information Is Giving Out, Communication Is Getting Through." oncnursingnews. Retrieved November 13, 2023, from https://www..com/view/information-is-giving-out-communication-is-getting-through

(Page 253) (n.d.). quotefancy. Retrieved November 14, 2023, from https://quotefancy.com/quote/117589 6/Albert-Ellis-Being-assertive-does-not-mean-attacking-or-ignoring-others-feelings-It-means

(Page 257) Rivenbark, C. (2023, November 15). celia-rivenbark-okay-lets-see-if-i-got-this-straight-the-butt-is-the-new-breast. theysaidso. Retrieved November 15, 2023, from https://theysaidso.com/quote/celia-rivenbark-okay-lets-see-if-i-got-this-straight-the-butt-is-the-new-breast

(Page 259) Cruz, G. (2023, June 18). "50 Inspirational Quotes For Organ Donation: Gift Of Life, Inspiring Generosity." letslearnslang. Retrieved November 15, 2023, from https://letslearnslang.com/inspirational-quotes-for-organ-donation/

(Page 263) Osler, W. (1999, May 17). https://www.azquotes.com/quotes/topics/probability.html. azquotes. Retrieved November 19, 2023, from https://www.azquotes.com/quotes/topics/probability.html

(Page 265) "Remembering Jim Rohn: 17 Remarkable Quotes to Inspire You." (2019, December 16). Retrieved November 21, 2023, from https://www.jimrohn.com/remembering-jim-rohn-17-remarkable-quotes-to-inspire-you/

(Page 267) Emily Ratajkowski Quotes . (n.d.). All Great Quotes. Retrieved November 27, 2023, from https://www.allgreatquotes.com/quote-125319/

(Page 271) Uitti, J. (2022, February 15). Top 22 Jim Morrison Quotes. American Songwriter. Retrieved December 1, 2023, from https://americansongwriter.com/top-22-jim-morrison-quotes/

(Page 276) Frost, M. (2016, September 6). Here's to the crazy ones. Mike Frost. Retrieved June 27, 2024, from https://mikefrost.net/heres-to-the-crazy-ones/

(Page 279) "Abu Bakr: 'Knowledge is the life of the mind.'". (n.d.). The Socratic Method. Retrieved January 2, 2024, from https://www.socratic-method.com/quote-meanings/abu-bakr-knowledge-is-the-life-of-the-mind

(Page 281) Dutta, M. (2023, December 12). "100 Skin Care Quotes To Help You Look After Your Body." Kidadl. Retrieved April 17, 2024, from https://kidadl.com/facts/quotes/skin-care-quotes-to-help-you-look-after-your-body

(Page 284) Vironitka Tugaleva Quotes. (n.d.). quote fancy. Retrieved April 18, 2024, from https://quotefancy.com/quote/3362089/Vironika-Tugaleva-Plenty-of-people-will-think-you-re-crazy-no-matter-what-you-do-Don-t

(Page 287) McCauley, T. (n.d.). "Do Not Reward Yourself With Food... You Are Not A Dog." The Gracious Pantry. Retrieved January 6, 2024, from https://www.thegraciouspantry.com/do-not-reward-yourself-with-food-you-

(Page 291) Druce, M. (2023, January 27). "Breast Cancer Quotes from Breast Cancer Warriors – 100+ Inspirational Quotes." The Breslow Center. Retrieved January 7, 2024, from https://breslowmd.com/breast-cancer-quotes/

(Page 292) Liles, M. (2023, January 9). "100 Funny Things To Say When You Want To Make Someone's Day." Parade. Retrieved January 8, 2024, from https://parade.com/1219273/marynliles/funny-things-to-say/

(Page 295) (n.d.). AZ Quotes. Retrieved January 9, 2024, from https://www.azquotes.com/quote/638731

(Page 297) Druce, M. (2023, January 27). "Breast Cancer Quotes from Breast Cancer Warriors – 100+ Inspirational Quotes." The Breslow Center. Retrieved January 9, 2024, from https://breslowmd.com/breast-cancer-quotes/

(Page 298) Milton, G. (2023, December 5). "50 Funny Weight Gain Quotes for Your Amusement and Motivation." collaborateforhealthyweight.org. Retrieved January 9, 2024, from https://collaborateforhealthyweight.org/funny-weight-gain-quotes/

(Page 301) Lauren, R. (n.d.). Ralph Lauren Quotes. AZ Quotes. Retrieved June 27, 2024, from https://www.azquotes.com/author/8547-Ralph_Lauren

(Page 303) Quote of the Day. (n.d.). Quoteslyfe. https://www.quoteslyfe.com/quote/Genetic-code-is-a-divine-writing-11496

(Page 305) Sweatshirt Jokes. (n.d.). UpJoke. Retrieved January 26, 2024, from https://upjoke.com/sweatshirt-jokes

(Page 307) "Watch out. Bras are often booby-trapped.". (n.d.). Quote Fancy. Retrieved January 26, 2024, from https://quotefancy.com/quote/77499/Tiffany-Reisz-Watch-out-Bras-are-often-booby-trapped

(Page 311) Bologna, C. (2023, November 9). "55 Funny Tweets About Hallmark Christmas Movies." Huff Post. Retrieved January 29, 2024, from https://www.huffpost.com/entry/hallmark-christmas-movies-funny-tweets_l_5fbdbc28c5b6e4b1ea46c3b4

(Page 318) Fell, J. S. (2018, September 25). "10 things we learned from Jack LaLanne." Chatelaine. Retrieved January 31, 2024, from https://chatelaine.com/health/fitness/10-things-we-learned-from-jack-la lanne/

(Page 321) Quotes. (n.d.). Good Reads. Retrieved February 3, 2024, from https://www.goodreads.com/author/quotes/89950.Ted_Zeff

(Page 325) "Quote Origin: Every Minute You Are Angry, You Lose Sixty Seconds of Happiness." (2023, March 18). Quote Investigator. Retrieved February 5, 2024, from https://quoteinvestigator.com/2023/03/ 18/minute-happiness/

(Page 328) Kate, G. (2023, May 10). "Negative Self Talk Quotes." The Goal Chaser. Retrieved February 6, 2024, from https://thegoalchaser.com/negative-self-talk-quotes/

(Page 332) (n.d.). AZ Quotes. Retrieved February 6, 2024, from https://www.azquotes.com/quote/565190

(Page 336) Olivia Newton-John. (n.d.). AZQuotes.com. Retrieved June 28, 2024, from AZQuotes.com Web site: https://www.azquotes.com/quote/565190

(Page 338) Mellina, C. (n.d.). Workcation. Alightthoughts. Retrieved February 7, 2024, from https://alignthoughts.com/jobs-fill-your-pocket-but-adventures-fill-your-soul/

(Page 340) Marr, D. (n.d.). AZ Quotes. Retrieved February 13, 2024, from https://www.azquotes.com/quote/548974

(Page 342) "50 Motivational Quotes About Weight Loss and Healthy Living." (n.d.). Inspirationalfeed. Retrieved February 13, 2024, from https://inspirationfeed.com/weight-loss-quotes/

(Page 346) Newsonen, S. (2018, June 20). "I Said to My Body: "I Want to Be Your Friend." Psychology Today. Retrieved February 14, 2024, from https://www.psychologytoday.com/us/blog/the-path-passionate-happiness/201806/i-said-my-body-i-want-be-your-friend

(Page 352) Winfrey, O. (n.d.). AZ Quotes. Retrieved February 16, 2024, from https://www.azquotes.com /quote/318151

(Page 357) Tracing Quotations. (2020, December 24). Quote Investigator. Retrieved February 17, 2024, from https://quoteinvestigator.com/2020/12/24/gift-life/

(Page 359) Demarco, C. (2018, December 12). "Best of Cancerwise 2018: 9 inspiring quotes from our cancer patients and caregivers." MD Anderson Center. Retrieved February 17, 2024, from https://www.mdanderson.org/cancerwise/best-of-cancerwise-2018--9-inspiring-quotes-about-cancer-treatment-and-survivorship.h00-159229668.html

(Page 363) Kacha, D. (n.d.). "Cancer Treatment Quotes." goodreads. Retrieved February 19, 2024, from https://www.goodreads.com/quotes/tag/cancer-treatment

(Page 365) Loving Mother and Son Quotes with the Deep Meaning (n.d.). Kind You. Retrieved February 20, 2024, from https://www.kindyou.com/loving-mother-and-son-quotes/

(Page 374) Vogel, K. (2020, February 3). "150 Inspiring Quotes on Beating Cancer from Super Survivors." Parade. Retrieved February 24, 2024, from https://parade.com/1140135/kaitlin-vogel/cancer-quotes/

(Page 379) Parkerton, M. (2023, March 22). "At a Loss For Words? Here Are 100 Thoughtful Messages to Write in a Get-Well Card for Cancer Patients." Parade. Retrieved February 26, 2024, from https://parade.com/1319349 /michelle-parkerton/get-well-wishes-for-cancer-patients/

(Page 384) Seltzer, L. F. (2014, November 2). "Wittiest Sex Quotes Ever." Psychology Today. Retrieved March 4, 2024, from https://www.psychologytoday.com/us/blog/evolution-the-self/201411/wittiest-sex-quotes-ever

(Page 388) Williams, T. T. (n.d.). Terry Tempest Williams Quotes About Cancer. AZ Quotes. Retrieved March 6, 2024, from https://www.azquotes.com/author/15727-Terry_Tempest_Williams/tag/cancer

(Page 391) Seybold, M. (2019, June 28). "THE APOCRYPHAL TWAIN: "THE THINGS YOU DIDN'T DO." Center For Mark Twain Studies. Retrieved March 6, 2024, from THE APOCRYPHAL TWAIN: "THE THINGS YOU DIDN'T DO."

CITATIONS FOR RESEARCH

(Page 8) "Getting Called Back After a Mammogram." (2022, May 17). American Cancer Society. Retrieved March 20, 2024, from https://www.cancer.org/cancer/types/breast-cancer/screening-tests-and-early-detection/mammograms/getting-called-back-after-a-mammogram.html

(Page 11) "Breast biopsy." (2023, August 25). Mayo Clinic. Retrieved March 20, 2024, from https://www.mayoclinic.org/tests-procedures/breast-biopsy/about/pac-20384812

(Page 16) Lewis, S. (2020, January 29). "Step-by-Step: What to Expect After a Breast Cancer Diagnosis." Treating Breast Cancer Early. Retrieved March 20, 2024, from https://www.healthgrades.com/right-care/breast-cancer/step-by-step-what-to-expect-after-a-breast-cancer-diagnosis

(Page 21) Wright, P. (n.d.). "Invasive Ductal Carcinoma" (IDC). Health. Retrieved March 22, 2024, from https://www.hopkinsmedicine.org/health/conditions-and-diseases/breast-cancer/invasive-ductal-carcinoma-idc

(Page 25) "Lumpectomy (Partial Mastectomy)." (2023, July 20). Web MD. Retrieved March 22, 2024, from https://www.webmd.com/breast-cancer/lumpectomy-partial-mastectomy

(Page 28) "Family and Medical Leave" (FMLA). (n.d.). U.S. Department of Labor. Retrieved March 22, 2024, from https://www.dol.gov/general/topic/benefits-leave/fmla

(Page 30) "What you should know and what you should ask about breast cancer." (2020, October 12). City of Hope. Retrieved March 22, 2024, from https://www.cancercenter.com/community/blog/2020/10/questions-breast-cancer

(Page 32) "Early Cancer Warning Signs: 5 Symptoms You Shouldn't Ignore." (n.d.). John Hopkins Medicine. Retrieved March 22, 2024, from https://www.hopkinsmedicine.org/health/wellness-and-prevention/early-cancer-warning-signs-5-symptoms-you-shouldnt-ignore

(Page 36) "Lymph node removal surgery (lymphadenectomy)." (2023, April 7). City of Hope. Retrieved March 23, 2024, from https://www.cancercenter.com/treatment-options/surgery/lymph-node-removal-lymphadenectomy

(Page 37) Burford, M. (2023, January 30). "Post-Lumpectomy Care Guide." verywellhealth. Retrieved March 24, 2024, from https://www.verywellhealth.com/post-lumpectomy-care-6822845

(Page 42) Jaber, N. (2021, January 14). "Study Suggests a Link between Stress and Cancer Coming Back." NATIONAL CANCER INSTITUTE. Retrieved March 24, 2024, from https://www.cancer.gov/news-events/cancer-currents-blog/2021/cancer-returning-stress-hormones

(Page 45) WebMD Editorial Contributors. (2023, October 24). "Tips for Recovering From Breast Cancer Surgery." WcbMD. Retrieved March 25, 2024, from https://www.webmd.com/breast-cancer/post-surgery-tips-breast-cancer

(Page 51) "Spiritual Support When You Have Cancer." (2022, September). Cancer.Net. Retrieved March 25, 2024, from https://www.cancer.net/coping-with-cancer/physical-emotional-and-social-effects-cancer/spiritual-support-when-you-have-cancer

(Page 54) Charly, A. T. (n.d.). "Answers by verified professionals." Ask a health professional. Retrieved March 26, 2024, from https://microsoftstart.msn.com/en-us/health/ask-professionals/in-expert-answers-on-breastcancer/in-breastcancer?questionid=k6s4soks&type=condition&source=bingmainline_conditionqna

(Page 56) OncoLink Team. (2024, March 8). "The Oncotype® DX Breast Recurrence Score." OncoLink. Retrieved March 26, 2024, from https://www.oncolink.org/cancers/breast/screening-diagnosis/the-oncotype-R-dx-breast-recurrence-score

(Page 63) Chemotherapy for breast cancer (2022, October 6). MayClinicRetrieve June 18, 2022 from https://www.mayoclinic.org/tests-procedures/chemotherapy-for-breast-cancer/about/pac-20384931#:~:text=Chemotherapy%20for%20breast%20cancer%20uses%20drugs%20to%20target,treatments%2C%20such%20as%20surg

(Page 68) Collins, V. W., & Gilliam, T. (2024). https://unclineberger.org/wp-content/uploads/sites/867/2018/09/CONDENSED_Lymphedema_ASelfCareGuide.pdf. UNC Health Care. Retrieved March 26, 2024, from https://unclineberger.org/wp-content/uploads/sites/867/2018/09/CONDENSED_Lymphedema_ASelfCareGuide.pdf

(Page 71) "Lymphatic Drainage Massage." (2021, September). Cleveland Clinic. Retrieved March 27, 2024, from https://my.clevelandclinic.org/health/treatments/21768-lymphatic-drainage-massage

(Page 72) "Is glaucoma related to cancer?" (2019, October 15). Quick-Advice. Retrieved March 27, 2024, from https://quick-advices.com/is-glaucoma-related-to-cancer/

(Page 74) "Obesity and lymphedema: Is there a connection?" (2023, May 23). Medical News Today. Retrieved March 27, 2024, from https://www.medicalnewstoday.com/articles/obesity-and-lymphedema

(Page 77) Veazey, K. (2021, August 24). "What to know about compression sleeves for lymphedema." Medical News Today. Retrieved March 29, 2024, from https://www.medicalnewstoday.com/articles/compression-sleeves-for-lymphedema

(Page 80) MD Anderson. (2014, September 17). "19 ways to help someone with cancer." MD Anderson Center. Retrieved March 29, 2024, from https://www.mdanderson.org/cancerwise/19-ways-to-help-someone-with-cancer.h00-158911701.html

(Page 84) "Should You Go on Vacation When Being Treated for Cancer?" (2021, January 7). Cleveland Clinic. Retrieved March 29, 2024, from https://health.clevelandclinic.org/should-i-go-on-vacation-when-im-being-treated-for-cancer

(Page 87) "Breast Cancer Can Be Genetic: Here's What To Know." (2024, March 25). Cleveland Clinic. Retrieved March 30, 2024, from https://health.clevelandclinic.org/is-breast-cancer-hereditary

(Page 90) Eldridge, L. (2022, May 21). "The Risk of Suicide in Cancer Patients." verywellhealth. Retrieved March 30, 2024, from https://www.verywellhealth.com/the-risk-of-suicide-in-cancer-patients-2248817

(Page 94) "Drinking Alcohol." https://give.breastcancer.org/give/294499/#!/. (2023, October 12). BreastCancer.Org. Retrieved April 1, 2024, from https://www.breastcancer.org/risk/risk-factors/drinking-alcohol

(Page 96) "Seroma formation after surgery for breast cancer." (2004, September). World Journal of Surgical Oncology. Retrieved April 1, 2024, from https://wjso.biomedcentral.com/articles/10.1186/1477-7819-2-44

(Page 98) "Brachytherapy." (2022, November 3). Cleveland Clinic. Retrieved April 1, 2024, from https://my.clevelandclinic.org/health/treatments/16500-brachytherapy

(Page 100) Web MD Editorial Contributors. (2024, March 13). "How Do Opioid Pain Meds Cause Constipation?" WebMD. Retrieved April 1, 2024, from https://www.webmd.com/pain-management/constipation-from-opioids

(Page 103) "Brachytherapy to Treat Cancer." (2019, January 29). National Cancer Institute. Retrieved April 2, 2024, from https://www.cancer.gov/about-cancer/treatment/types/radiation-therapy/brachytherapy

(Page 106) "Komen Financial Assistance Program." (n.d.). Susan G. Komen. Retrieved April 2, 2024, from https://www.komen.org/financial-assistance-program/

(Page 108) Purse, M. (2024, March 19). "Valium to Manage Anxiety Disorders and Symptoms." Verywell mind. Retrieved April 3, 2024, from https://www.verywellmind.com/valium-drug-information-380681

(Page 111) Pure Wow. (2020, April 29). "An Easy Way to Waterproof Your Phone So You Can Run in the Rain." yahoo! life. Retrieved April 3, 2024, from https://www.yahoo.com/lifestyle/easy-way-waterproof-phone-run-012800800.html?guccounter=1&guce_referrer=aHR0cHM6Ly93d3cuYmluZy5jb20v&guce_referrer_sig=AQAAAGh-OLTfr9BWg2q_tarQGEdd7j---kCiREzF_X4R_5Vc3

(Page 112) Nolan-Pleckham, M. (2022, August 27). "10 Pillows to Use for Comfort During Breast Cancer Treatment and Recovery." Verywell health. Retrieved April 3, 2024, from https://www.verywellhealth.com/comfort-pillows-breast-cancer-recovery-430551

(Page 115) Editorial Team. (2021, November 8). "Breast Cancer Grade." American Cancer Society. Retrieved April 3, 2024, from https://www.cancer.org/cancer/types/breast-cancer/understanding-a-breast-cancer-diagnosis/breast-cancer-grades.html

(Page 118) "Radiation Therapy to Treat Cancer." (n.d.). National Cancer Institute. Retrieved April 3, 2024, from https://www.cancer.gov/about-cancer/treatment/types/radiation-therapy

(Page 120) Fordyce, K. (2023, March 17). "Breast Cancer and Your Sex Life." Web MD. Retrieved April 3, 2024, from https://www.webmd.com/breast-cancer/breast-cancer-sex-life

(Page 126) Rutherford, G. (2020, June 3). "Bell ringing ritual to mark end of cancer treatment builds community, gives patients a sense of control, study finds." Medical X press. Retrieved April 4, 2024, from https://medicalxpress.com/news/2020-06-bell-ritual-cancer-treatment-patients.html

(Page 130) Jones, B. (2022, April 26). "Fatigue During Cancer Radiation Therapy." very well health. https://www.verywellhealth.com/fatigue-and-radiation-therapy-514353

(Page 132) Program Finder. (n.d.). "Look good feel better." Retrieved April 4, 2024, from https://lookgoodfeelbetter.org/programs/program-finder/

(Page 135) Ohio State University. (2020, June 3). "A satisfying romantic relationship may improve breast cancer survivors' health." ScienceDaily. Retrieved April 4, 2024 from www.sciencedaily.com/releases/2020/06/200603194436.htm

(Page 136) Ferrara, N. B. (2022, January 19). "Regaining sexual health after cancer treatment." Mayo Clinic Comprehensive Cancer Center BlogNews, information and stories from Mayo Clinic's cancer experts and patients. Retrieved April 4, 2024, from https://cancerblog.mayoclinic.org/2022/01/19/regaining-sexual-health-after-cancer-treatment/

(Page 140) "Male Breast Cancer – What you need to know." (n.d.). Male Care. Retrieved April 4, 2024, from https://malecare.org/male-breast-cancer/

(Page 145) Drisdelle, D. (n.d.). "How to Plan for Air Travel with Lymphedema." flow lymphatic health clinic. Retrieved April 5, 2024, from https://lymphatichealthclinic.com/how-to-plan-for-air-travel-with-lymphedema/

(Page 149) Carter, K. (2023, March 28). "New Meanings and Shifting Priorities." Surviving Breast Cancer. Retrieved April 5, 2024, from https://www.survivingbreastcancer.org/post/new-meanings-and-shifting-priorities

(Page 154) Conner, K., & DePolo, J. (n.d.). "Returning to Work After Breast Cancer Treatment." https://give.b. BreastCancer.org. Retrieved April 5, 2024, from https://www.breastcancer.org/managing-life/cancer-survivorshi p/returning-to-work-after-cancer

(Page 156) Ramshaw, W. (2022, January 15). "6 Ways to Stop Worrying About Your Cancer Returning and Live Your Life." Cure. Retrieved April 6, 2024, from https://www.curetoday.com/view/6-ways-to-stop-worrying-about-your-cancer-returning-and-live-your-life

(Page 159) Cleveland Clinic. (2022, June 29). "Inflammatory Breast Cancer." Cleveland Clinic. Retrieved April 6, 2024, from https://my.clevelandclinic.org/health/diseases/17925-inflammatory-breast-cancer

(Page 164) Letrozole Tablets. (n.d.). Cleveland Clinic. Retrieved April 6, 2024, from https://my.clevelandclinic .org/health/drugs/18808-letrozole-tablets

(Page 165) City of Hope. (2019, December 26). "The power of laughter for cancer patients." City of Hope. Retrieved April 6, 2024, from https://www.cancercenter.com/community/blog/2019/12/power-of-laughter-for-cancer-patients

(Page 168) Sissons, B. (2022, November 17). "Can hormonal imbalances cause depression?" Medical News Today. Retrieved April 6, 2024, from https://www.medicalnewstoday.com/articles/hormonal-depression#:~:text=A%20drop%20in%20hormones%20can,depression

(Page 172) "Celebrate Being Cancer Free: 10 Ideas from a Breast Cancer Survivor" (2023, July 26). Life After Cancer. Retrieved April 6, 2024, from https://www.mycancerchic.com/ways-to-celebrate-being-cancer-free/

(Page 177) Madormo, C. (2021, December 19). "Why are Cancer Patients at Increased Risk for Infection?" very well health. Retrieved April 6, 2024, from https://www.verywellhealth.com/risk-for-infection-and-cancer-5210860

(Page 180) "Deciphering Your Lab Report." (2021, January 27). Testing. Retrieved April 7, 2024, from https:/ /www.testing.com/articles/how-to-read-your-laboratory-report/

(Page 184) eHealthMe. (2024, February 5). "Will you have Urinary tract infection if you take Letrozole?" eHealthMe. Retrieved April 7, 2024, from https://www.ehealthme.com/ds/letrozole/urinary-tract-infection/

(Page 186) Levofloxacin. (2023, October 4). Drugs.com. Retrieved April 7, 2024, from https://www.drugs.com/levofloxacin.html

(Page 187) DePolo, J. (n.d.). "COVID-19: What People Diagnosed With Breast Cancer Need To Know." Breast Cancer. Org. Retrieved April 7, 2024, from https://www.breastcancer.org/managing-life/staying-well-during-covid-19/what-people-with-breast-cancer-need-to-know

(Page 192) "What Does That Mean? — Glossary." (n.d.). rethink Breast Cancer. Retrieved April 8, 2024, from https://rethinkbreastcancer.com/glossary/(Page 195) Why MD Anderson. (n.d.). MD Anderson Center. Retrieved April 8, 2024, from https://www.mdanderson.org/patients-family/becoming-our-patient/why-md-anderson.html

(Page 200) Shafqat, H. (2023, November 16). "How Cancer Patients Can Boost Their Immune System." Bens Natural Health. Retrieved April 8, 2024, from https://www.bensnaturalhealth.com/blog/how-cancer-patients-can-boost-immune-system/

(Page 206) "Does Letrozole Cause Weight Gain?" (2022, August 7). Breast Cancer 101. Retrieved April 8, 2024

(Page 207) Livestrong Voices. (2018, May 15). Four Things You Should Know about LIVESTRONG at the YMCA. Medium. Retrieved April 9, 2024, from https://blog.livestrong.org/four-things-you-should-know-about-livestrong-at-the-ymca-94f41515dc1f

(Page 209) "Goal setting during your cancer journey." (n.d.). Piedmont. Retrieved April 9, 2024, from https://www.piedmont.org/living-real-change/goal-setting-during-your-cancer-journey

(Page 211) "How Surgery Affects the Immune System https://give.breastcance. (2024, January 8). Breast Cancer. org. Retrieved April 9, 2024, from https://www.breastcancer.org/managing-life/immune-system/cancer-treatments/surgery

(Page 213) Scott, J. (2023, August 30). "Can altering cancer 'mindsets' change physical outcomes?" Scope. Retrieved April 9, 2024, from https://scopeblog.stanford.edu/2023/08/30/can-altering-cancer-mindsets-change-physical-outcomes/

(Page 218) Medicare Made Clear. (n.d.). "How often should a woman over 65 have a Pap smear?" United Health Care. Retrieved April 9, 2024, from https://www.uhc.com/news-articles/medicare-articles/how-often-should-a-woman-over-65-have-a-pap-smear

(Page 219) Editorial Board. (2021, March). "Weight Gain." Cancer.Net. Retrieved April 10, 2024, from https://www.cancer.net/coping-with-cancer/physical-emotional-and-social-effects-cancer/managing-physical-side-effects/weight-gain

(Page 221) "Physical Activity and Cancer." (n.d.). National Cancer Institute. Retrieved April 11, 2024, from https://www.cancer.gov/about-cancer/causes-prevention/risk/obesity/physical-activity-fact-sheet

(Page 226) Ferrara, N. B. (2022, December 6). Why you should ask about cancer clinical trials. Mayo Clinic Comprehensive Cancer Center BlogNews, information and stories from Mayo Clinic's cancer experts and patients. Retrieved April 11, 2024, from https://cancerblog.mayoclinic.org/2022/12/06/why-you-should-ask-about-cancer-clinical-trials/

(Page 231) Scott, J. (2023, February 8). "See an Oncologist." verywellhealth. Retrieved April 12, 2024, from https://www.verywellhealth.com/how-to-survive-cancer-513771

(Page 235) Herndon, J. (2018, September 17). "What Is a Transvaginal Ultrasound?" healthline. Retrieved April 14, 2024, from Transvaginal Ultrasound: Purpose, Procedure, and Results (healthline.com)

(Page 237) "12 Powerful Uterine Cancer Symptoms." (2019, January 13). veryhealthy life. 12 Powerful Uterine Cancer Symptoms (veryhealthy.life)

(Page 240) Fernandez, S. M. (1998, July). "Pretty in Pink." History of the Pink Ribbon. Retrieved April 15, 2024, from History of the Pink Ribbon - Breast Cancer Action (bcaction.org)

(Page 243) "Adjustment to Cancer: Anxiety and Distress (PDQ®)–Patient Version." (2023, June 23). National Cancer Institute. Retrieved April 15, 2024, from https://www.cancer.gov/about-cancer/coping/feelings/anxiety-distress-pdq

(Page 246) "Aromatase Inhibitor Treatment And Weight Gain" | Food for Breast Cancer. (2022, June 11). Foods for Breast Cancer. Retrieved April 15, 2024, from https://foodforbreastcancer.com/articles/aromatase-inhibitor-treatment-and-weight-gain

(Page 250) "How to Ask for Clarification." (2019, January 3). Everyday Grammar. Retrieved November 13, 2023, from https://learningenglish.voanews.com/a/how-to-ask-for-clarification/4726030.html

(Page 252) (2021, April 15). "MEDICAL TREND." Retrieved November 14, 2023, from 5-year cancer survival rate: Can cancer patient only live for 5 years?

(Page 257) "5 Things You Might Not Know About Breast Implants." (n.d.). blackdoctor.org. Retrieved November 14, 2023, from https://blackdoctor.org/breast-implants-risks__trashed/

(Page 259) Swenson, K. (2023, June 13). "AlloDerm: What You Need to Know." realself. Retrieved November 15, 2023, from https://www.realself.com/surgical/alloderm

(Page 262) "Breast Cancer by State: How Different States Rank in Breast Cancer Mortality Rates." (2023, September 20). National Breast Cancer Foundation, Inc.. Retrieved November 15, 2023, from https://www.nationalbreastcancer.org/blog/breast-cancer-by-state-how-different-states-rank-in-breast-cancer-mortality-rates/#:~:text=Based%20on%20nationwide%20breast%20cancer%20incidence%20and%20death

(Page 265) Vogal, K. (2021, October 15). "A Rash Can Be a Symptom of Breast Cancer—Here Are the Top Signs to Look Out for if You're Worried You Have One, and When to See a Doctor." Parade. Retrieved November 21, 2023, from https://parade.com/1276573/kaitlin-vogel/breast-cancer-rash/

(Page 267) "6 Swimsuit Brands for Breast Cancer Thrivers!" (n.d.). Rethink Breast Cancer. Retrieved November 27, 2023, from https://rethinkbreastcancer.com/6-swimsuit-brands-for-breast-cancer-thrivers/

(Page 270) Gesualdi-Gilmore, L. (2020, February 22). "Cancer Ghosting' Is Real — Many Survivors Say Friends Suddenly Disappear After a Diagnosis." Survivornet. Retrieved December 1, 2023, from https://www.survivornet.com/articles/cancer-ghosting-is-real-many-survivors-say-friends-suddenly-disappear-after-a-diagnosis/

(Page 276) "Hormone Balancing." (n.d.). Pacific Brain Health Center. https://www.pacificneuroscienceinstitute.org/brain-health/diagnostics-procedures/hormone-balancing/

(Page 279) "Exemestane 25 Mg Tablet Aromatase Inhibitors - Uses, Side Effects, and More." (n.d.). Web MD. Retrieved January 2, 2024, from https://www.webmd.com/drugs/2/drug-17764/exemestane-oral/details

(Page 280) Schiff, T. (2021, October 28). "The Surprising Link Between Breast Cancer and Skin Cancer." Water's Edge Dermatology. Retrieved January 2, 2024, from https://www.wederm.com/2021/10/28/the-surprising-link-between-breast-cancer-and-skin-cancer/

(Page 284) Grace J Yoo: Ellen G Levine: Caryn Aviv: Cheryl Ewing: Alfred AU. (2009, November). "Older women, breast cancer, and social support." PMC PubMed Central. Retrieved April 18, 2024, from https://www.ncbi.nlm.nih.gov/pmc/articles/PMC2959163/

(Page 287) "15 Cancer Fighting Foods." (2019, January 9). Very Healthy Life. Retrieved January 6, 2024, from https://veryhealthy.life/15-cancer-fighting-foods/?utm_source=foods%20that%20help%20fight%20cancer&utm_medium=15CancerFightingFoods&utm_campaign=adw_us&msclkid=c5ad92bcaeba16996921f7268cf5757b

(Page 291) "My breast implants are leaking — Health risks?" (n.d.). Go Ask Alice. Retrieved January 7, 2024, from https://goaskalice.columbia.edu/answered-questions/my-breast-implants-are-leaking-health-risks/

(Page 292) "Intrusive Thoughts Are All in Your Head." (2023, July 14). Cleveland Clinic. Retrieved January 8, 2024, from https://health.clevelandclinic.org/intrusive-thoughts

(Page 294) "After breast reconstruction: what to expect." (n.d.). Breast Cancer Now The research & support charity. Retrieved January 8, 2024, from https://breastcancernow.org/about-breast-cancer/treatment/surgery-for-primary-breast-cancer/breast-reconstruction/after-breast-reconstruction-what-to-expect/

(Page 296) "CAPSULAR FIBROSIS WITH BREAST IMPLANTS." (n.d.). theaesthetics. Retrieved January 9, 2024, from https://www.theaesthetics.at/en/capsular-fibrosis-with-breast-implants/

(Page 298) "8 Unforeseen Reasons For Weight Gain After Surgery." (2023, January 12). Health Guide. Retrieved January 9, 2024, from https://healthguidenet.com/conditions/weight-gain-after-surgery/

(Page 301) Nunez, K. (2020, January 28). "What's It Like to Recover from Breast Augmentation Surgery?" Healthline. Retrieved January 24, 2024, from https://www.healthline.com/health/breast-augmentation-recovery

(Page 303) "Does DNA Get Washed Out Over Generations?" (n.d.). What are you made of. Retrieved January 24, 2024, from https://whoareyoumadeof.com/blog/does-dna-get-washed-out-over-generations/

(Page 305) "Doctor humour: 15 health specialist who know how to have a laugh" (n.d.). The Wonderlist. Retrieved January 26, 2024, from https://thewonderlist.net/doctor-humour-15-health-specialist-who-know-how-to-have-a-laugh/

(Page 306) Weil, A. (2014, October 21). "Do Bras Cause Breast Cancer?" Weil. Retrieved January 26, 2024, from https://www.drweil.com/health-wellness/body-mind-spirit/cancer/do-bras-cause-breast-cancer/

(Page 311) "Hallmark Keepsake Ornament." (n.d.). Susan G. Komen. Retrieved January 29, 2024, from https: //www.komen.org/how-to-help/support-our-partners/hallmark/

(Page 318) Wark, C. (n.d.). "How I used the Raw Vegan Diet to Beat Cancer." Chris Beat Cancer. Retrieved January 31, 2024, from https://www.chrisbeatcancer.com/the-raw-vegan-diet/

(Page 320) Howley, E. K. (n.d.). Why Is Fear Such a Problem With Breast Cancer? U.S. News. Retrieved February 3, 2024, from https://health.usnews.com/health-care/patient-advice/articles/2017-10-31/why-is-fear-such-a-problem-wit h-breast-cance

(Page 325) "Common Errors in Medical Billing and Coding and How to Avoid Them." (2018, May 17). MTI College. Retrieved February 5, 2024, from http://mticolleges.weebly.com/blog/common-errors-in-medical-billing-and-coding-and-how-to-avoid-them

(Page 328) Seladi-Schulman, J. (2021, November 16). "How Much Does Medicare Part B Cost?" healthline. Retrieved February 5, 2024, from https://www.healthline.com/health/medicare/medicare-part-b-cost#:~:text=If%20you%20have%20Part%20B%2C

%20you%E2%80%99ll%20need%20to,known%20as%20an%20income-related%20monthly%20adjustment%20amount%20%2

(Page 331) Gordon, S. (2019, July 17). https://consumer.healthday.com/cancer-information-5/mis-cancer-news-102/can-a-broken-heart-contribute-to-cancer-. Health Day. Retrieved February 6, 2024, from https://www.healthday.com/health-news/cardiovascular-diseases/can-a-broken-heart-contribute-to-cancer-748387.html

(Page 335) "10 ways to celebrate your cancerversary." (2017, October 25). Endeavor Health. Retrieved February 6, 2024, from https://www.eehealth.org/blog/2017/10/10-ways-to-celebrate-your-cancerversary/

(Page 338) "Emotion and care." (2023, November 9). National Cancer Institute. Retrieved February 7, 2024, from https://www.cancer.gov/about-cancer/coping/feelings

(Page 339) Laird, P. B. (2021, June 4). "Cancer-Causing Chemicals in Sunscreens? Here's What You Need to Know." Resource Blog From Baptist Health South Florida. Retrieved February 13, 2024, from https://baptisthealth.net/baptist-health-news/cancer-causing-chemicals-in-sunscreens-what-you-need-to-know

(Page 342) Rosen, N. S. (2023, January 19). "With growing popularity of new weight loss drugs, doctors emphasize potential risks." abc News. Retrieved February 13, 2024, from https://abcnews.go.com/Health/growing-popularity-new-weight-loss-drugs-doctors-emphasize/story?id=96424302

(Page 343) Darrisaw, M. (2019, January 16). "In My Humble Opinion, Loofahs Are More Disgusting Than Washcloths—And Doctors Agree." Oprah Daily. Retrieved February 14, 2024, from https://www.oprahdaily.com/life/a25893661/loofah-vs-washcloth/

(Page 346) Simran, . (n.d.). "Body Dysmorphic Disorder: Signs, Causes, Treatment And More." Mantra Care. Retrieved February 14, 2024, from https://mantracare.org/therapy/what-is/body-dysmorphic-disorder/

(Page 351) "The Best (and Worst) Ways to Support a Friend With a Serious Illness." (n.d.). Healthy Tips. Retrieved February 16, 2024, from https://www.nm.org/healthbeat/healthy-tips/emotional-health/the-best-and-worst-ways-to-support-a-friend-with-a-serious-illness

(Page 354) Whitney, C. M. (2012, October 22). "Celebrating Healthy Birthdays." Integrative Oncology Essentials. Retrieved February 17, 2024, from https://integrativeoncology-essentials.com/2012/10/celebrating-healthy-birthdays/

(Page 358) Eldridge, L. (2021, September 7). "Coping With Scanxiety During Cancer Treatment." verywell health. Retrieved February 17, 2024, from https://www.verywellhealth.com/coping-with-anxiety-waiting-for-test-results-3955875

(Page 363) Cafasso, J. (2021, May 4). "Is Breast Cancer Curable? Get the Facts." healthline. Retrieved February 19, 2024, from https://www.healthline.com/health/breast-cancer/breast-cancer-cure

(Page 365) Edwards, B. (2014, February 17). "'GOD, IF YOU…THEN I'LL…': WHY YOU CAN'T BARTER WITH GOD." DETROIT BAPTIST THEOLOGICAL SEMINARY. Retrieved February 20, 2024, from https://dbts.edu/2014/02/17/god-if-youthen-ill-why-you-cant-barter-with-god/

(Page 370) "Surprising Things That Can Help During and After Breast Cancer Treatment." (2023, October 24). WebMD. Retrieved February 21, 2024, from https://www.webmd.com/breast-cancer/ss/slideshow-surprising-breast-cancer-help

(Page 374) "Not As You Know It." Retrieved February 24, 2024, from https://metro.co.uk/2018/02/03/why-is-cancer-called-cancer-7284242/

(Page 379) Eldridge, L. (2022, October 20). Reducing the Risk of Breast Cancer Recurrence. Verywellhealth. Retrieved February 26, 2024, from https://www.verywellhealth.com/reducing-breast-cancer-recurrence-4688612

(Page 383) "How Cancer and Cancer Treatment Can Affect Sexuality." (n.d.). American Cancer Society. Retrieved March 3, 2024, from https://www.cancer.org/cancer/managing-cancer/side-effects/fertility-and-sexual-side-effects/how-cancer-affects-sexuality.html

(Page 388) Marcus, M. B. (2015, October 19). HEALTH "Are the kids all right? When breast cancer runs in the family." Health. Retrieved March 6, 2024, from https://www.cbsnews.com/news/breast-cancer-genes-family-history-impact-on-girls/

(Page 391 Kember, L. (2023, March 6). "Vacation Cruise Can Soothe Cancer Patient, Caregiver." Abestos.com. Retrieved March 6, 2024, from https://www.asbestos.com/blog/2013/10/15/cancer-patient-caregiver-vacation-cruise/

www.ingramcontent.com/pod-product-compliance
Lightning Source LLC
Chambersburg PA
CBHW040003040426
42337CB00033B/5207